The Alarming H

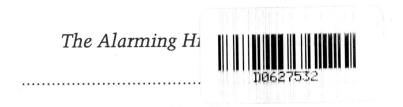

D0627532

By the same author

RICHARD GORDON

The Alarming History of Medicine

St. Martin's Griffin
New York

THE ALARMING HISTORY OF MEDICINE.
Copyright © 1993 by Richard Gordon Ltd.
All rights reserved. Printed in the United States of America. No part
of this book may be used or reproduced in any manner whatsoever
without written permission except in the case of brief quotations
embodied in critical articles or reviews. For information, address
St. Martin's Press, 175 Fifth Avenue, New York, N.Y. 10010.

Library of Congress Cataloging-in-Publication Data

Gordon, Richard.
The alarming history of medicine : amusing anecdotes from
Hippocrates to heart transplants / Richard Gordon.
p.   cm.
ISBN 0-312-16763-6
1. Medicine—Anecdotes.   2. Therapeutics—Anecdotes.
I. Title.
R705.G648   1994
610-dc20   93-37558   CIP

First published in Great Britain by Sinclair-Stevenson Limited.
First St. Martin's Griffin Edition: October 1997

10   9   8   7   6   5   4   3   2   1

The tragedy of man is that he has developed an intelligence eager to uncover mysteries, but not strong enough to penetrate them.

Hans Zinsser *Rats, Lice and History*

The philosophies of one age have become the absurdities of the next, and the foolishness of yesterday has become the wisdom of tomorrow; through long ages which were slowly learning what we are hurrying to forget, amid all the changes and chances of twenty-five centuries, the profession has never lacked men who have lived up to the Greek ideals.

Sir William Osler *Aequanimitas and Other Addresses*

Just think of it. A hundred years ago there were no bacilli, no ptomaine poisoning, no diphtheria, and no appendicitis. Rabies was but little known, and only imperfectly developed. All of these we owe to medical science. Even such things as psoriasis and parotitis and trypanosomiasis, which are now household names, were known only to the few and were quite beyond the reach of the great mass of the people.

Stephen Leacock *How to be a Doctor*

Contents

List of Illustrations

1 The first transplant: saintly surgery by Cosmas and Damian.
   Alonso de Sedano – The Trustee of The Wellcome Trust, London.
2 Vesalius teaching anatomy.
   The Trustee of The Wellcome Trust, London.
3 Domicilliary delivery, sixteenth century.
   Edinburgh University Library.
4 Doctor's plague kit.
   The Trustee of The Wellcome Trust, London.
5 Weight watching, 1614.
   The Trustee of The Wellcome Trust, London.
6 A touch of royalty: Charles II's TB clinic.
   The Trustee of The Wellcome Trust, London.
7 Hogarth's doctors, sniffing their gold-headed canes and tasting their patients' urine.
   The Trustee of The Wellcome Trust, London.
8 Juptile and the mad dog in the Institut Pasteur, Paris.
   Institut Pasteur.
9 Europe's first anaesthetic. Liston is performing the operation (on the wrong leg).
10 Lord Lister's carbolic spray.
   Guthrie, D., A History of Medicine.
11 The father of medicine, Hippocrates.
   British Museum.

The Alarming History of Medicine

ONE

Hippocrates and All That

The history of medicine is not the testament of idealistic seekers after health and life; no more than the history of man is more glorious than a catalogue of selfish and brutish unreason shot spasmodically with sanity.

The history of medicine is largely the substitution of ignorance by fallacies. Such wandering up blind alleys can be a useful progression, if the more intelligent and impatient stragglers reconnoitre a better way. 'Many remarkable discoveries have been achieved by men, who, following the traces of nature with their own eyes, pursued her through devious but most assured ways till they reached her in the citadel of truth,' it was put by the man who discovered the circulation of the blood.

About every generation since 1600, these individualists have bestowed upon mankind some biological boon unrelated to the bleak progress of its conventional benefactors. That their discoveries were generally beset with unsuspected perils, causing unexpected disease and death, only adds to the excitement of the story.

The hewers of extensions to this vale of tears are a rum lot: all clever, some cunning, the lucky ones anointed with inspiration or serendipity, many of them simply abnormally obsessive classifiers of men and microbes, or simply abnormally deft-fingered. Their academic caps buzzed with bees which sometimes honeyed the bread of affliction. They mingled with illusionists. Medicine has persistently decked itself out in fashions shamming achievements, while staying miserably bare on masterly discoveries. These make a round dozen, which are listed at the end of the book for the intelligent reader to test his or her perceptiveness.

(The intelligent reader having got so far standing in the library or bookshop, may feel that turning them up now will save further trouble and some expense.)

Here Be Dragons

The early history of medicine is immensely boring. Egyptian Imhotep (c 2980 BC) combined the convenience of physician and monumental mason for Pharaoh Zoser, by building the magnificent Step Pyramid of Sakkarah, for the gracious use of his royal patient when he had passed beyond treatment. Chinese Emperor Fu-Hsi (c 2900 BC) would today be a fashionable practitioner of alternative medicine, pricking his acupunctures and directing the bodily flow of Yang and Yin. These are the opposing forces of life and death, of male and female, of strength and weakness, of sun and moon. Yang wallows in the bloody heart and lungs, Yin resounds in the hollow bowels and bladder. What curiously enduring nonsense! Emperor Huang Ti (c 2650 BC) discovered the circulation of the blood 4278 years before William Harvey – if he existed at all, emperors waft through the rarefied air of Chinese history like the dragons. In their mingled history and legends, perhaps the ancient Chinese inoculated against smallpox through blowing its dried pustule crusts up the nose. Perhaps they really fed cretin children, who suffered from deficient thyroids, with the thyroid gland butchered from sheep. Perhaps they enjoyed cannabis, employed blind masseurs and were keen on cold baths, and perhaps they could diagnose all diseases from subtle study of the pulse. It is all too remote for our excitement, and too occult for our tuition. Our only certainty is that the ancient Chinese, like the mass of mankind before the nineteenth century, mostly lived and died with only the therapeutic botheration of traditional and futile sorcery. Happily, man had always the poppy to benumb, the grape to soothe.

The Greeks substituted for Yang and Yin the humours. Blood, phlegm, yellow and black bile, your health depended on their harmony at the moment. The top Greek doctor was Galen (c AD 131–200). He was an overbearing man with the answer to everything, so setting one persistent personality pattern in our profession. He observed that the arteries contained blood, not air. He was an expert on wounds (surgeon to the gladiators) and foreshadowed transplants by noticing that the heart still beat when cut from its body (at sacrifices). The dictatorship of his dogma ruled medicine for fifteen centuries: in 1559, Henry VIII's Royal College of Physicians was carpeting an Oxford man who dared to suspect his infallibility.

Galen practised among the Romans, who considered professional medicine *infra dignitatem*. Their Celsus (c AD 50) was a nobleman and gifted amateur doctor, flattered in literature as the *Cicero medicorum*. His elegant encyclopaedia *De Medicina* enjoyed the everlasting distinction of joining the first printed books in 1478.

3

Celsus instructed on the operations for hernia and tonsil-lectomy ('to be disengaged all round by the finger and pulled out'), he glimpsed the shadows looming across mankind of *insania* and *cardiacus*, he anticipated Harvey (in partnership with the Emperor Huang Ti) with his fleeting intuition *sanguis cursus revocetur*, and he provided us with the signs of inflammation *calor, rubor, tumor, dolor*. Enough Latin.

Charaka, Susruta, Alcmæon, Empedocles, Pythagoras and Aristotle are distant stars twinkling in the outer space of medical history but unnecessary to magnify.

Hippocratic Time-bomb

Everyone knows Hippocrates (460–370 BC). This is because of his Oath, which few doctors can recite, or even recall beyond a friendly discouragement to avoid sex with their patients. The Oath's embellishing *Precepts* warn practitioners against overcharging, overdressing and wearing perfume, while urging upon them a decent haircut and trimming the nails, and encouraging the assumption of a pleasing bedside manner (the term was bestowed by *Punch* in 1884).

As Watt invented the steam-engine, Hippocrates invented clinical medicine. It is a simple mechanism: the practical application of intelligent observation. It is the sick man who matters, not man's theories of sickness. And the entire patient must be heeded, his whole surroundings noticed – holistic medicine, twenty-one centuries before it became faddish.

Hippocrates' firsts:

– He laid ear to chest to catch the friction of the inflamed membranes in pleurisy, which sounded to him like the creaking of new leather.

- He was struck by the sharp-nosed, hollow-eyed, cold-eared face of impending death, the *Hippocratic facies* worn by Falstaff in *Henry V*, when 'his nose was as sharp as a pen and a' babbled of green fields'.
- He had pondered over a dying man's strange breathing since his case of 'Philiscus, who lived by the wall, and took to bed on the first day of acute fever . . . about the middle of the sixth day he died. The respiration throughout like that of a man recollecting himself, and rare, and large.'

    These famous last gasps resurfaced in 1818 in Dublin. John Cheyne (1777–1836) wrote about a case of apoplexy: 'For several days his breathing was irregular; it would entirely cease for a quarter of a minute, then it would become perceptible, though very low, then by degrees it became heaving and quick, and then it would gradually cease again. This revolution in the state of his breathing occupied about a minute.' Twenty-eight years later, William Stokes (1804–78) fished it out again for medical Dublin's attention, these two *émigré* Scotsmen's names to be linked evermore in 'Cheyne-Stoking' – from a failing respiratory centre in the brain – the head-shaking professional harbinger of doom.
- Hippocrates spotted that tar (an antiseptic) stopped suppuration in wounds. He drained pus, aligned fractures and popped back dislocations.
- He established the principle: 'Our natures are the physicians of our diseases.' Which means, that most people get better anyway.

Hippocrates was born on the Greek island of Cos, off Turkey, and taught under a plane tree (viewable, to tourists). He gave us the word 'aphorism'. He uttered 412. As:

Life is short, the art is long. (A depressing chiselling over the entrances to medical schools.)
Opportunity is fleeting, experiment dangerous,

judgment difficult. (Equally so.)

Desperate cases need desperate remedies.

Old people endure fasting best, next the middle-aged, youths badly and worst of all children. (Hence a fortune in middle-aged diet books.)

Do not judge the stool by its quantity but by its quality. ('Twice round the pan and pointed at both ends,' was sadly misplaced perfectionism in an old country doctor.)

Sleep that ends delirium is good; undue sleep and sleeplessness indicates disease; so does unprovoked tiredness.

The old are ill less than the young but carry their illnesses to the grave.

Sudden death is commoner in the fat than the thin.

If a healthy woman stops menstruating and feels sick she is pregnant. (We all know all these things. But it was Hippocrates who knew them first.)

The 'Father of Medicine' was a disastrous ancestor. He left the Hippocratic tradition. This is, shortly: any non-doctor telling a doctor how to do his job is committing outrageous impertinence; any interference with the wherewithal for any doctor's selfless devotion to his patients is shockingly immoral.

Hippocrates would have been baffled by the appearance of Plato announcing that he was the Cos Area Health Authority. Even Marcus Aurelius would have hesitated stepping down from the Capitol and telling Galen that his budget was being cut. *Eheu fugaces!* By the end of the twentieth century, medicine has so proliferated, and its costs have so escalated, that serious treatment is far beyond the means of the frightened sufferers, and will eventually be beyond those of any state's suffering tax-payers. Unless doctors learn to practise economics as well as medicine, Hippocrates will be made redundant because nobody will be able to afford being ill.

Hippocrates shines fancifully in the gallery of ancient

medical statuary, curly-bearded and furrowed-browed over the ills of mankind (viewable in the British Museum). He often bears the serpent-twined staff of Aesculapius, the God of Healing. On rowdy and confusing Olympus, Aesculapius was the son of Apollo (doctor to the gods) and Coronis (nymph). He was so effective a practitioner that he annoyed Pluto by dwindling the population of Hades, so Zeus exploded him with a thunderbolt. He is viewable in the Tate Gallery, in Sir Edward Poynter's 1880 portrait of Aesculapius' clinic: a walled garden atinkle with fountains and acoo with doves, his patients four voluptuous stark naked girls, plump in bosom and mons veneris, the only evident sufferer presenting the doctor with a troublesome heel to her left foot. Lucky old Aesculapius.

Hippocrates wrote 100 books, though he was as plausibly as Shakespeare a committee.

The Unpopularity of Death

Timor mortis conturbat me – the thought of dying scares me to death, exclaimed William Dunbar (?1465–?1530), the Scottish Chaucer, if such a transmigration is possible. This reasonable foreboding created religion and the medical profession.

The early Christian Church resented doctors. They interfered in the death business. The corpses nestled round its ivy-mantled tow'rs emphasised that Heaven's welcome for its patrons would be as warm as Hell's chastisement of the rest. The cause of disease was obviously sin, its treatment was prayer, fasting and repentance. The saints ran the body. St Blaise had charge of the throat, St Bridget the eyes and St Erasmus the guts, St Dympna was the psychiatrist, St Lawrence specialised in backache, St Fiacre in the sore arse (he gave his name to the French cab). St Roche distributed the plagues, St Vitus had his dance, St Anthony's Fire roasted the limbs, ignited either by infection or the poison of ergot-infected rye bread. The first transplant operation was performed by the saintly twins, Cosmas and Damian, who replaced the ulcerated leg of a white man with the black one from a newly-dead Moor (de Sedano got the picture). They were decapitated in AD 303, for being unorthodox nuisances.

Worse, the human corpse was held sacred beyond dissection (the Moslems went along with this). So knowledge of the body remained skin-deep.

Galen grumbled that a physician without anatomy was an architect without a plan, but even he had to make do with dissecting the Barbary apes now embellishing the Rock of Gibraltar. Trotula (c 1050) was one of the obstetrical 'ladies of Salerno' (the others were Abella, Constanza and Rebecca), she was the author of *De Mulierum Passionibus*, she was renowned in song as 'Dame Trot' from Navarre to Paris by famed *trouvère* Rutebœuf, but she still had to dissect pigs. She comforted herself by reasoning that they looked like men inside. Across the Mediterranean, at the Alexandria medical school founded in 332 BC, Herophilus and Erasistratus (c 300 BC) already had the anatomical answer: they dissected criminals from the royal prison, alive. 'By far the best method for attaining knowledge,' Celsus recorded approvingly.

Anatomy was dead, and medicine stillborn. Religion is of course a Good Thing, offering the valuable incidentals of saddling assertive man with someone more important than himself, giving a set of excellent rules on which, by and large, he fails to run his life, affording him hope, comfort, guidance and humility, and providing some delightful architecture from St Peter's to the Taj Mahal. But it scuppered healing for fifteen centuries.

Leonardo da Vinci (1452–1519) was a casual anatomist. The Queen keeps at Windsor his delightful drawing of a sliced couple having sex. They use the standing position, and present in longitudinal section the penis firmly in vagina, with stout nerves transmitting the fun to the man's spinal cord, his heart pumping the semen out of his scrotum through a long spinal tube, and her uterus plumbed to her nipple. The accompanying detail of a penis sliced like a saveloy displays correctly its spongy caverns, which flood on erection with blood. Though the adjoining illustration of the female genitalia imparts a robustness matching the entrance to a cathedral. It is all a reasonable conception of events.

Paris medical student Andreas Versalius (1514–64) encountered outside the walls of Louvain, near his native Brussels, a gibbet still swinging with a desiccated skeleton *complete with ligaments*. He hurried home his prize – any human skeleton was a *rara avis* – to found a career which culminated with a crammed anatomical amphitheatre in Padua (Titian got the picture). The artistry of Versalius' lovely anatomical atlas *De Humani Corporis Fabrica* gives the flayed bodies, their muscles opening like blooming petals, the springing vivacity of Wimbledon tennis-players. He bravely debunked Galen, after discovering that the jaw was one bone not two, the breastbone three bones not seven, and that the sons of Adam had no missing rib, so Eve must have come from somewhere else. All of which incurred the ageless wrath of people who think themselves important.

Heresy and blasphemy persisted as pompous guises for suppressing free speech, the object of which always implicitly affords the suppressors secret uneasiness. Even Pope Urban VIII must have stirred in his sleep wondering if, perhaps, Galileo was possibly right, and *eppur si muove.* Michael Servetus (1509–53) was burned alive by Calvin for discovering the pulmonary circulation, his books fuelling his flames. Versalius was forced to abandon anatomy aged thirty, and took the job of court physician in Madrid. He dissected a Spanish nobleman, who alarmingly stirred under the knife, which incurred the wrath of the Inquisition, who sentenced him to an expiating trip to Jerusalem, on which he was shipwrecked and died of hunger in the Greek island of Zante. After Versalius came Eustachius (1510–74) and Fallopius (1523–62), famous for their tubes (one in the middle ear, the other in the female pelvis).

Dame Trot's Salerno in the eleventh century was the first medical 'centre of excellence', a term now applied to themselves by Guy's, Bart's, Tommy's etc. This popular seaside spa became the original *Civitas Hippocratica*, a meeting place for doctors in delightful surroundings on tax-free expenses. Napoleon shut the medical school in 1811. It is no longer viewable, like the rest of old Salerno after the bombardment for the Allied landings on 9 September 1943.

Salerno was superseded in excellence during the thirteenth century by Montpellier, and then by Leyden medical school near The Hague, which was founded by William of Orange in 1575. Leyden's star was Hermann Boerhaave (1668–1738), a practical physician who lectured elegantly in Latin, drew students even from America, had a private practice extending to China, and left two million florins. Montpellier fleetingly nourished drunken, wandering, quarrelsome, arrogant Paracelsus (1493–1541) from Zurich, who began his lectures by burning copies of Galen, and disdained medical traditionalists, his contemporaries, physicians' velvet robes and uttering Latin. 'I pleased no one except the sick whom I healed,' he boasted applaudably. Montpellier produced the only medical Pope, John XXI, who died when his ceiling fell on him.

Sixty-five years after Versalius became its professor of anatomy and surgery, Padua educated William Harvey (1578–1657) from Folkestone, who was short, swarthy, curly-haired, jumpy and talkative, and went home to become physician at St Bartholomew's Hospital and to James I and Charles I.

Everybody knew that the blood moved, from the spurting artery of a slaughtered sheep, or from men's baffling propensity for killing and wounding each other (Harvey always wore a dagger at his belt). Until the seventeenth century, everybody imagined it went in and out, like the tides. In 1628, Harvey showed it went round and around, like the 1930s music.

There was a sticking point: how did blood return to the pumping heart through the unyielding flesh? Galen had said it shuttled from one side of the heart to the other. 'We are driven to wonder at the handiwork of the Almighty,' commented Versalius sarcastically, 'by means of which the blood sweats from the right into the left ventricle through passages which escape the human vision.' The answer tantalised Harvey's students for thirty-two years.

The microscope was accidentally invented by a Dutch optician getting two lenses stuck in a tube. Antony van Leeuwenhoek (1632–1723) of Delf exploited it – he had 247 of them, and was the first man to see his spermatozoa. The microscope of Marcello Malpighi (1628–94) in Bologna displayed Harvey's missing link, by showing the whole body honeycombed with minute capillary bloodvessels which channelled the arteries to the veins. Henceforth, the body was as joyfully microscoped as anatomised all over Europe.

Our body is the same old body as primitive man's. It springs the same old diseases. Our skulls are still those which ancient well-wishers, with painful logic, bored holes in to relieve headaches or release the devils of madness. Mummies suffered appendicitis, arthritis and bad teeth. (For mummification, you insert a hook through the nose to extract the brain, slice open the flanks and draw like oven-ready poultry, stuff with spices and pickle in salt for seventy days.) Even dinosaurs had bad backs.

Corpses were the common-land on which medicine grazed and fattened. Supplies were philanthropically ensured by criminals, for whom their gruesome dissection became a sharper deterrent than the preceding hanging. When stock ran short at Edinburgh for scintillating lecturer Robert Knox (1791–1862), Burke and Hare could always dig up someone to help. This couple's trouble was laziness. To save shadowing funerals, evading watchful relatives in the dark, and digging hurriedly with wooden tools to dampen the noise, they stupefied live bodies with whisky, strangled them, and sacked 'em up at £7.10s apiece. 'Resurrectionists' were rife, until the British Anatomy Act of 1832 substituted filling in a form by visionary volunteers. There was a terrible row in Montreal in 1875, when typhoid hit a convent school and the nuns and children were filched before the American parents arrived to bring home the corpses.

Anatomists have carved their names on us as lovingly as sweethearts on trees. We contain the crypts of Lieberkühn, in the lining of the intestines. The circle of Willis, which is a joining of arteries at the base of the brain. The ampulla of Vater, guarding the end of the bile duct. The foramen of Winslow, a hole in the abdominal lining below the liver. The fossa of Rolando in the brain, and the sheath of Schwann on the nerves. The pouch of Douglas behind the uterus, Alcock's canal in the pelvis ('Not the vagina', pun medical students). Bell's nerve in the chest, Santorini's muscle on the face, Poupart's ligament in the groin, Scarpa's triangle on the thigh . . . You find it, you name it. This exuberant egotism has left us glorious walking Pantheons to the greatest doctors of five centuries. And why not?

The physicians meanwhile obliged the Church by searching for the soul, but even Sir Thomas Browne of Oxford, Montpellier, Padua and Leyden Universities failed to find it. René Descartes (1596–1660) who promoted *l'homme-machine* (man was a *deux-chevaux*, God its Maker, with Holy Spirit in the tank) located the soul in the pineal gland, a teardrop behind the main ventricle of the brain. Nobody knows what the pineal gland does, but it may make us feel happier in bright sunshine, so he was probably right.

William Harvey wrote in *Exercitatio Anatomica de Motu Cortis et Sanguinis in Animalibus*:

> It may very well happen thus in the body with the movement of the blood. All parts may be nourished, warmed and activated by the hotter, perfect vaporous, spirituous and, so to speak, nutritious blood. On the other hand, in parts the blood may be cooled, thickened, and be figuratively worn out. From such parts it returns to its starting point, namely the heart, as if to its source or to the centre of the body's economy, to be restored to its erstwhile state of perfection. Therein, by the natural, powerful, fiery heat, a sort of store of life, it is reliquified and becomes impregnated with spirits and (if I may so style it) sweetness. From the heart it is redistributed. And all these happenings are dependent upon the pulsatile movement of the heart

13

Today, this is put:

ELECTRICAL EXCITATION OF THE HEART
Working myocardium (Non-pacemaker cells)
Changes in membrane potential:
Phase 4
Resting potential (-90 mV)
Near K-equilibrium potential.

Scientifically if depressingly, we are but waterproof bags of electrically charged chemicals, which one day befall a power failure. So are our dogs, the birds in the garden, the elephants in the zoo, the mice in the kitchen, the goldfish, the greenfly on the roses, the single-celled amoeba which gives us dysentery, the flu virus. Unlike them, unlike even the apes swinging from the branches immediately below us in the evolutionary tree, we know that we shall die.

'This body is not, cannot be, all that I am – that is the human cry,' recognised C. P. Snow. Thus mankind conceived the life eternal, from a mixture of fright and vanity. And God became a happy human creation, like Mickey Mouse.

'Where there are three physicians there are two atheists,' said the Latin medieval proverb. Though any doctor would be pleasantly surprised to reawake on a cloud playing a harp with Bertrand Russell, who philosophised steadfastly: 'When I die I shall rot,' for ninety-seven years before he did.

TWO

Man, Microbes and History

The summer of 1894 was terrible in Woking. The Martians had landed. They were the size of bears, oily-skinned, with two huge eyes, and slavering mouths be-whiskered with bunches of whippy tentacles. They never ate – they had no entrails – but injected human blood into their veins. They never slept nor even felt tired. They went 'Ulla, ulla, ulla, ulla!' and reproduced by budding. They spread an entangling carpet of red weed, and emitted fatal heat rays and black poison gas. The invaders advanced up the seemly Chobham road and took demure Byfleet, despite the Hussars and the Maxims. Weybridge fell, Shepperton was devastated, the population of London fled to Barnet. The Martians continued their murderous way to Primrose Hill, where they all caught something and died. They had conquered man, but they embodied no resistance whatever to the bacteria which teemed across man's Earth. Our germs delivered us. The germs did for the red weed, too.

The War of the Worlds

At H. G. Wells' birth in 1866, nobody knew the Earth's army of microbes existed. At his death in 1946, we were attacking it into patchy submission. The meek micro-organism inherited the earth before us, they infinitely outnumber us, they stealthily murder us, they rein our sexual delights, they piloted our history and commanded our wanderings, they intermittently massacred us, they reduce us to pitiable fright and ludicrous finicalness, they are fragile, flexible, irrepressible and invincible, they will be here after us. Their discovery in the second half of the last century was a materialisation of the goblins, gnomes, elves, imps and leprechauns frolicking timelessly in our folk memory. It's a bugs' world.

The thirteenth chapter of Leviticus is a masterly hand-book of public health. For the control of leprosy, the sufferer's clothes are burnt – whether warp or woof, in woollen or in linen – and crying 'Unclean, unclean!' he vanishes into isolation. Couples with gonorrhea face quarantine for a week, everything they sat on to be washed, including their saddles. Man ever knew that he could catch an illness from someone or from something – but only vaguely, as he still imagines the chill wind to blow him rheumatics. Even Hippocrates failed to twig on to infection.

Fever was accorded to the gods, or more specifically to bad air – *malaria* expresses the Italian shiver at poison-ous emanations from the Pontine Marshes. It took the devastating plagues of the Middle Ages to rouse desperate suspicion that something *solid* must transmit disease from one of us to another. In 1546, a jovial physician and poet from Verona, Hieronymus Fracastorius (1483–1553), pondered in *De Contagione* that the epidemics which slew on the shores of Lake Garda progressed by unseen seeds. These seeds were swiftly propagating, wafted by breath or by the air, or by drinking from the same cup or lying with the same woman, by clothes, combs, coins, anything infected, what he called 'fomites'. He failed only to grasp that the seeds were living, as he was.

Nothing much else happened in the conquest of infection until 17 September 1683.

Our bustling draper from Delft, Antony van Leeuwenhoek, was as fashionable a creator of microscopes as his contemporary Stradivarius was of violins. That September day, he picked his teeth and discovered little animals 'more numerous than the population of the Netherlands, all moving about delightfully.' These were bacteria, in their now familiar and typical clumps and chains. These 'animalcules' persisted in the medical mind as being generated, like maggots, by the putrefying flesh itself. As insects to the Chinese were supposedly engendered by damp bamboo, bees arose from dead cows, and the sunbaked Nile mud gave birth to frogs and snakes, if not alligators.

When Francesco Redi (1626–97) of Tuscany anticipated Mrs Pooter by covering the meat to keep out the flies, he abolished the maggots. They did *not* sprout spontaneously. *Omne vivum ex ovo*, he announced, even a grub has a mum and dad. Only Homer had the idea before:

'Mother,' complained Achilles at Troy, 'I am terribly afraid meanwhile that flies may defile the corpse of my lord Patroclus by settling on the open wounds and breeding worms in them.'
'My child,' Thetis comforted him, 'I will arrange to

17

keep away the flies and save him from those pests that devour the bodies of men killed in battle.'

Mother Thetis' preventative treatment was ambrosia and red nectar, given through the nostrils.

Fashions in doctoring recur as sillily as in dress designing. Those maggots which crawled so repulsively around wounds were doing nothing but good. They were hungrily clearing away the septic debris of dead skin and flesh and pus, and are now facing recruitment as nontoxic body scavengers. For an external aural infection, nothing is better than a maggot in your earhole.

Nobody got significantly further until the arrival of the nineteenth century's greatest doctor, who was unqualified.

Pasteurised Medicine

In 1856, the French wine industry was corked. Bottle after vinegary bottle was angrily returned to *sommeliers*, disgustedly poured into the sewers, despairingly smashed against the walls. The beer was pretty nasty, too. The frenzied vintners of Bordeaux sent for the Professor of Chemistry at Lille, as reputable an authority on fermentation as Flaubert in nearby Rouen on adultery.

Louis Pasteur (1822–95) from the Jura was the son of a tanner, who was a veteran of *la grande armée*. Pasteur in 1864 found this tragic acidification of wine to be perpetrated not by malignant chemistry, but by living microscopic organisms, generated not by the agreeable fluid itself, but dropping upon it from the air. The œnological disaster was preventable by killing the organisms, through heating the vat to 60° C. These vintages so *bien chambrées* were gulped with such joyful relief, the French wine industry rocketed to a 500 million francs yearly turnover. Pasteur then saw that the yeasts of good beer were spherical, of bad beer elliptical, a distortion caused by microbes. So he Pasteurised the beer, too.

The French silk industry was meanwhile plummeting from a 130 million to an 8 million francs annual income, because the silkworms had all caught *pébrine*, black pepper disease. Silkworms love mulberries, but the plantations of mulberry bushes in the Cévennes Mountains of Languedoc had alarmingly become vermiculite ghost towns. In confused desperation, the sericulturists sought Pasteur.

He went south from Paris to Alais, and rewarded them by discovering the silkworm epidemic to be inflicted by some sort of living microbe (it was a protozoan, a single-cell organism like the amoeba which gives you dysentery, but for the moment he was unable to put his hands on it). Pasteur threw in another disease, *flâcherie*, silkworm diarrhoea. The cures for both were culling the insects which showed the peppery spots – the peasants bottled the silkworm moths in brandy, for display to the experts – and rigorous hygiene of the mulberry leaf. Soon the rustle of silk is heard in our land.

It is comforting to reflect that the genesis of anaesthesia lay in the vapour-sniffing 'ether frolics', and that of bacteriology – with its benevolent offshoots of inoculation and antibiotics – in a glass of wine, a jug of beer and a pretty dress. Our instincts for enjoying ourselves have vindicatory side-effects.

The cows and sheep of France were having a bad time, too. They were being decimated by anthrax, extremely painfully. In 1881, Professor Pasteur's anti-anthrax vaccine reduced the mortality of this disease to 1 per cent in sheep and 0.34 per cent in cattle. The chickens all got cholera. Pasteur happened to forget on his laboratory bench a specimen of the bacterial fluid which infected the chickens, and went on holiday. He returned to discover this culture of growing bacteria was weakened, and found it ideal for inoculation against the pestilence – like another holiday, we shall see, in a bleaker climate, let the penicillin mould grow perfectly for Alexander Fleming. How clever to win the Nobel Prize *in absentia*.

From the marrow of the spines of mad dogs Pasteur grew a vaccine which saved the life of shepherd-boy Juptille, now forever bravely battling with a rabid dog in the 15th *arrondissement*. He embellishes the courtyard of the Institut Pasteur, where lies entombed our conceiver of living microbes, and of scientific inoculation to combat their unceasing campaigns against us.

Pasteur's mind was the light at the end of the infective tunnel that had no beginning. The cash value of his discoveries to France were reckoned to balance the indemnity exacted by Germany for the war of 1870–71. He lived simply, seriously and spiritually, and did it all despite suffering a disabling stroke in 1868. His twelve-year-old daughter died of typhoid fifteen years before the typhoid germ was discovered. The application of his genius to milk in the twentieth century created Pasteur a doorstep name in Britain.

Method in their Microbes

In 1771, sensible Dr Tobias Smollett could forthrightly summarise:

> Snares are laid for our lives in every thing we eat or drink: the very air we breathe, is loaded with contagion. We cannot even sleep, without risque of infection.

Frenchman Louis Pasteur enlightened the medical profession that the mysterious infective 'things' which passed diseases were living things. Classifying the precise sorts of these things was an obstacle which the orderly German mind busily demolished.

On the other side in the 1870 war fought Robert Koch (1843–1910), a village GP at Wollstein in the Rhineland, who got bored with rough journeys and rustic patients and sought intellectual diversion down a microscope. He started by studying a hefty bacillus discovered in 1863 by Frenchman Casimir Davaine (1812–1882), who was otherwise a tapeworm specialist. With the unfussy eye of a country doctor, Koch observed the propensity of this bacillus for forming itself into endless chains, and its disappearance into long-living spores of lurking virulence. And that it caused anthrax.

This was the medical sensation of 1876. Robert Koch had linked germ to disease like cause to effect, a pathological marriage nobody had contemplated.

Anthrax in man or beast, with its bloody pustules on the skin, its swiftly lethal 'woolsorter's disease' of the lungs, had been shruggingly ascribed to the miasmas of the countryside. Koch proved anthrax to be an identifiable infection coming from an identifiable bug. Better still, he vividly dyed these invisible enemies, he learned what they liked to eat while they proliferated bountifully in captivity (cold beef *consommé*), he took dramatic photos of them. 'C'est un grand progrès!' he was greeted heartily in London by Pasteur, who went home to Paris to engineer the growth of the anthrax bacillus in an attenuated form, to make a vaccine to save the meat and cheese of France.

Koch propounded Koch's Postulates:

1 The germ causing a disease must be discoverable in all cases of the disease, and found in the body wherever the disease lies.
2 Extracted from the body, the germ must grow in a pure

laboratory culture, for several microbial generations. (Bacteria have no sex-life, they just go on splitting in two.)

3 This culture must give the disease to a susceptible animal, be recoverable from it in a pure culture, and transmit the disease to another unfortunate beast.

Such proof of a specific microbe causing a specific disease has remained watertight since its creation in 1881, precisely like the Mersey Tunnel.

In 1879, Albert Neisser (1855–1916), a Breslau dermatologist, discovered the gonococcus. And Armauer Hansen (1841–1912) of Bergen justified Leviticus by discovering the leprosy bacillus (Norway was becoming a leper nation). In 1880, Pasteur discovered the streptococcus and staphylococcus, which cause all sorts of infections. And Karl Joseph Eberth (1835–1926), a richly-bearded pathologist from Halle, discovered the typhoid bacillus. In 1882, Koch discovered the microbe causing tuberculosis. His later successor at his new Institute for Infectious Diseases, Friedrich Loëffler (1852–1915), that same year discovered the glanders bacillus, and the next, with testy Edwin Klebs (1834–1913) from Königsberg, the diphtheria bacillus.

Koch then discovered the cholera bacillus, in Berlin in 1884 Albert Fränkel (1848–1910) found the coccus which caused pneumonia, and Arthur Nicolaier (1862–?) discovered the tetanus bacillus. In 1886, goateed Theodor Escherich (1857–1911) from Munich identified the coli bacillus, which gets in everyone's guts. Running up the Union Jack, Sir David Bruce in 1887 discovered the microbe of Malta fever, while Anton Weichselbaum (1842–1920) in Austria discovered the one causing meningitis. In 1889, another Koch disciple, Richard Pfeiffer (1858–1945) at Breslau discovered the influenza bacillus, which unfortunately does not cause influenza. In 1892 fluttered the Stars and Stripes, when William Welch (1850–1934) discovered the armies' terror, the oxygen-despising bacillus of gas gangrene. And 1894 flew the Rising Sun, as fat Shibasaburo Kitasato (1852–1931), also a Koch man, with Frenchman Alexander Yersin (1862–?) discovered the germ that, by bringing bubonic plague, had bestowed terror upon the ages.

Eighteen years, and eighteen mass murderers tagged and corralled.

> O world invisible, we view thee,
> O world intangible, we touch thee,
> O world unknowable, we know thee,
> Inapprehensible, we clutch thee!

Bacteriologists could now proclaim ex-medical student Francis Thompson's (1859–1907) apostrophe to the spiritual life, but more usefully. Robert Koch won the Nobel Prize in 1905, his ashes lie in the Koch Institute in Berlin.

Probably Just a Virus

Mosaic disease smouldering in the tobacco plantations in 1892, and foot-and-mouth disease down on the farm in 1898, argued that some disorders could be transmitted without bacteria. You could pass them experimentally by an infective fluid, and this penetrated a filter impermeable to all the known microbes. The culprits were viruses, which reproduce (asexually, by binary fission) only inside living cells. They are smaller than bacteria and visible only to electron microscopes. Some are nothing more than protein-coated nucleic acid. Some are so simple they are capable of crystallisation: chemicals, but living things, like us. Perhaps thus we all started as scum upon the primeval slime.

Viruses menace us fellow-creatures with unpleasant and dangerous diseases, from poliomyelitis and pneumonia to colds and warts. We selfishly see ourselves as prime targets of the swarming, battle-thirsty, bacterial and viral army. But animals and fish, flowers and trees, insects and oysters, all have their health and lives endangered by infection. On the Swiftian principle that fleas have smaller fleas to bite 'em, even bacteria fall ill and die from the tiny tadpole-like bacteriophage viruses which were discovered in 1915. All of us live on something else. Our world is a parasitic paradise.

The Salmonella Show

So many species and subspecies of bacteria were being discovered under the sway of Queen Victoria and her grandson Kaiser William, they demanded classification in a microbial telephone directory. The motile, tail-waggling *Salmonella* group now embraces over 1000 different species causing gut infections. They entered everyday conversation and raised public and political panic in Britain in 1988, with the spectacular resignation of Under-Secretary of Health Edwina Currie (b 1946).

Man had then achieved through his enviable ingenuity microwave ovens and chilled food, which are ideal for the nourishment and propagation of his unseen unicellular enemies. And his comfortable air-conditioning had turned into a murderous menace a previously unconsidered coccobacillus, which now spreads Legionnaires' disease. Feeding chickens economically on their own droppings, rich with *Salmonellae*, had similarly transformed the egg of English breakfasts into lightly-boiled Borgias, driving English poultry farms towards the ruin of earlier French *vinicoles*. The founder classifier of *Salmonella* was Daniel Elmer Salmon (1850–1914), a distinguished-looking American thatched with white hair, with commanding eyebrows, a spruce moustache and a neat goatee. I was puzzled, after meeting him photographically in the Wellcome Medical Museum, what notable person this guru of gut-rot so strikingly resembled. Until encountering in the street outside his double, everybody's finger-licking friend, the sanitary saintly Colonel Saunders.

Plagues Upon Us

The German mentality sprang to the marshalling of microbes as agilely as to metaphysics or mysticism. The British one explored the diseases upon which the sun never set.

Hindu doctor Susruta (*c* AD 500) had suspected malaria to be inflicted not by the air, but instead by the mosquitoes which buzzed through the steamy twilight (as shrewdly as he suspected that a plethora of dead rats presaged the plague). Marco Polo in the thirteenth century had observed the mosquito-nets which later draped the dreams, the passions and the sweaty insomnia of the British Raj. Gowned Cambridge dons were struck by 'marsh fever' from the dank fens, but remained as imperceptive as everyone else of the villainous insect which injected such widespread intermittent ague. Until 6 November 1880, when a French Army MO posted to Algeria, Alphonse Laveran (1845–1922), discovered the single-cell *Plasmodium* parasite in the red blood corpuscles of malarial patients.

Scotsman Sir Patrick Manson (1844–1922) went forthrightly from Aberdeen University into the Chinese Imperial Maritime Customs Service, arriving on the beach at Formosa on a dark night in 1866. Three years before Laveran's discovery, he asserted in Hong Kong that the five centimetre-long filaria worm caused elephantiasis, a condition arising from blockage of the human lymph ducts, which can cause gigantic swelling of the limbs and necessitate the perambulation of the scrotum in a wheelbarrow. Further, he found that the minute, highly motile larval filaria worms, which teem in the patient's blood at night, were sucked up by the biting *Culex fatigans* mosquitoes, then incubated inside them, and then passed to someone else. Nobody believed this.

Manson came home and founded the London School of Tropical Medicine. In 1894 he met the future Sir Ronald Ross (1857–1932), India born, son of a general, bull-necked with a spiked NCO's moustache, just off the P & O liner on leave from the Indian Medical Service. Manson introduced Ross down the microscope to the French officer's Algerian malarial parasite. Keen Ross, back in his Calcutta lab opposite the statue of Queen Victoria, encountered this again on 20 August 1897, in the stomach of the *Anopheles* mosquito, which has spotted wings.

So jubilant was the British Empire at elucidation of the disease which devastated indiscriminately and impertinently the ruled natives and their sola-topied, fly-whisking rulers, this date became 'Malaria Day', with terrific annual lunches at the Ross Institute in Putney. Ross also wrote poetry, which appealed strongly to Osbert Sitwell. Another bacteriological poet was Max von Pettenkofer (1818–1901) of Bavaria, a Victor Hugo lookalike who shot himself. Von Pettenkofer disbelieved so fiercely in Koch's discovery of 1884 – that cholera was caused by a comma-like motile germ – that he publicly swallowed a contaminated glassful. He got away with it, unlike Tchaikovsky.

Sir Ronald Ross' theory was conclusively proved right by Manson, who set infected mosquitoes to bite a healthy young man, who developed malaria, who was his son. The Empire swiftly declared war upon the mosquito, devastating its landing grounds, felling it in flight, coating its targets with repellent lotions. The Americans, as on two other occasions, followed the Empire into the fight.

The French company which started digging the Panama Canal in 1880 went bankrupt in 1888. It had employed 86,800 men, of whom 52,816 fell sick and 5,627 died, mostly from yellow fever. This is an explosive jaundice, a virus disease transmitted by the tiger mosquito, which has stripes. Such was proved in the Manson tradition by two Baltimore bacteriologists, James Carrol (1854–1907) and Jesse Lazear (1866–1900), who were both bitten by infected mosquitoes. (Carrol recovered. Lazear died.)

The American tactician of the Canal war was Major Walter Reed (1851–1902), a bacteriologist from Johns Hopkins University, who had already swept the mosquito from Havana. His field commander was energetic Colonel William Crawford Gorgas (1854–1920) of Mobile, who had survved an enemy attack when serving as an army surgeon in Texas. Colonel Gorgas went into action with flame-throwers, hit-squads, chemical warfare, water-traps and fines for harbouring the enemy, all prisoners to be gassed by chloroform. His offensive was reckoned to cost the US $10 a mosquito. When the Canal was opened in 1913, the Canal Zone – going on the death rate – was more than twice as healthy as the United States.

The two centimetre-long brownish blood-sucking tsetse fly transmits sleeping sickness to man, from the reservoir of the disease in wild animals, by the sinuous long-tailed *Trypanosoma* protozoan. This was discovered in the blood of sufferers in 1894 by Sir David Bruce, after he had changed his outpost of Empire from Malta to Zululand. The tsetse fly was first noticed by David Livingstone (1813–73), ex-Glasgow mill-hand, doctor, missionary, explorer, discoverer of the grandiose Victoria Falls, sufferer for thirty years from an ununited fracture of the upper arm after a lion bite. He saw the fly in 1857, fourteen years before he got lost.

Today, one-third of the world's deaths are fly-related.

Febrifuge Fables

The paroxysms of malarial fever, every second or third day, express the time needed for the four different types of parasite to perform their asexual reproductive cycle in the blood. Their sexual cycle is enjoyed in the mosquito. Quinine, with its impressively bitter taste, was the malarial medicine since the seventeenth century. It was traditionally named 'cinchona' after the Countess of Chinchon, who was dispatched with her husband from Spain to Peru and was cured of malaria by the bark of the local quina-quina tree. The efficiency of the quina-quina was discovered by a fevered patient, the only drinking-water he could find being a pool into which these trees had been thrown, and was too bitter for the taste of the healthy. The Countess had the bark powdered and boun-tifully dispensed throughout Lima, before benevolently bestowing it on Spain. (The Countess died before her husband was posted to Peru as Viceroy, his accompany-ing second wife never suffered a day's illness, and she stayed out there, but good fiction is stranger than truth.) Imported 'Jesuit's bark', adulterated with any old wood, was henceforth snapped up by malarial Europe, except by Oliver Cromwell on religious grounds.

In World War Two, the British Empire could conveniently protect its soldiers with mepacrine, a drug which clever German chemists had evolved from the brilliant dyes they synthesised at Wuppertal in 1930. Word spread through the ranks, as it does about any compulsory medicine, that mepacrine caused impotence. The rumour of bromide in the soldiers' tea is as old as the story of the two Chelsea Pensioners admitting that it was beginning to take effect. This canard was countered by posters of pashas surrounded by their harems, gleefully taking the tablets and declaring they would never be without them. It seemed to satisfy the troops.

Now we have better anti-malarial prophylactics and better insecticides, but we still have malaria. We cannot extinguish every mosquito in up-country Thailand and Malaysia. And the parasites are getting wise to the drugs. Just like all those germs which were targeted by mankind in the 1880s.

Sunshine and Moonshine

The sun that shone uninterruptedly upon the British Empire occasioned the same continuing concern in Whitehall as the Devil in the Vatican. Englishmen clearly needed to go out in it – someone had to handle the mad dogs – but equally the *sahib* could not risk extinction by sun-stroke. 'Adequate protective covering for the head by thick pith topees or good cork helmets is essential,' the Empire's standard medical textbook was commanding in the year of the Battle of Alamein. 'Spinal pads for the protection of the spinal cord are valuable. Hand-fans and umbrellas are of value.' The Americans, having no Empire, went about Africa bare-headed. This encouraged General Montgomery's medical officers in the Desert campaign to junk the sola topi, so Hitler's spies peering past the pyramids accurately reported the reinforcements newly arriving from Britain by numbering the topied troops marching through the streets of Cairo.

This solar suspicion infected the Empire's favourite game. Accommodation in any mature English cricket pavilion today, as at Lord's itself, is bereft of sunshine. The rough workers opposite across the pitch were obliged to face the reasonable hazard of sun-stroke for cheap seats to watch the Test matches. At garden-parties and picnics Edwardian ladies muslinned and tuled themselves and twirled their parasols against such glaring inconvenience. Ladies then progressively removed all their clothes in the sunshine over the advancing century, and are frantically putting them all back on again. The wisdom of remaining deadly pale on holiday is now readily accepted, confronting the naked truth of the sun's skin malignancies.

Heat-stroke is inflicted not by sunlight but by salt deficiency. This was neatly illustrated by Sir Victor Horsley (1857–1916), the London brain surgeon who invented Horsley's wax for controlling skull haemorrhage. The wax was appropriately an adaptation of modelling wax, Horsley's father being a Royal Academician, who outrageously opposed nude artists' models. Sir Victor was equally condemnatory of tobacco and alcohol. He maintained fiercely that it was the lavish *chota* pegs and sundowners which caused sun-stroke, not venturing out without your sola topi. He proved this in Mesopotamia by going hatless, and shortly died of heat-stroke.

Stimulate the Phagocytes

'The physician of the future will be an immuniser,' brazenly prophesied Sir Almroth Wright (1861–1947), professor at the British Army Medical College in 1900, and friend of fellow Irishman George Bernard Shaw.

Shaw later came often to tea with Wright at the Innoculation Department of St Mary's Hospital in London. Shaw modelled phagocyte-stimulating Sir Colenso Ridgeon on him in *The Doctor's Dilemma*, from which Sir Almroth walked out of the first night in 1906.

The South African War of 1899–1902, the first tolling clang for the British Empire, was not won with the scratch rifles of Boer farmers, but by the typhoid bacillus. Of every thousand soldiers sent to the Cape it killed fifteen, twice as many as the enemy managed to. Sir Almroth Wright conceived inoculation, by injecting attenuated typhoid bacilli to create patients' resistance to the real thing. The Army scoffed. Sir Almroth quit. By World War One, the Army had time for the idea to sink in, and few died from typhoid, even at Gallipoli, where it thrived. The Army was inoculated against tetanus, too, which was liable to rub from the earth into wounds. This became a reduced hazard in World War Two, because tanks, unlike horses, do not defaecate.

The inoculated horse, with customary obligingness, produces voluminous anti-serum to combat the same germs as are slaughtering its masters. Against lobar pneumonia, this *passive* inoculation failed. Against a killer of the young, diphtheria, it worked. Diphtheria could have been abolished by *active* inoculation, like typhoid in the Army, after 1926. But nobody bothered much until 1940, so 50,000 civilians, more than in the Blitz, died unnecessarily of apathy.

Sir Almroth Wright at eighty had the humiliation of rescinding his young self-confidence. He confessed wretchedly to the Royal Society of Medicine about 'the need for abandoning much in immunology regarded as assured.' The sulpha drugs and penicillin were massacring the germs which he had so ingeniously turned upon themselves. He would have died happier, had he seen immunisation fired against the viruses of measles, of

German measles (with the menace to pregnancy), whooping cough, polio, hepatitis, and the same diseases he himself fought between the wars. Immunisation is back again. Germs can turn cleverly and savagely on their chemical attackers, and man is meddling with his immunology by intruding transplants.

The Itch to Kill

To terrorise us, our unicellular aggressors can evoke powerful allies. Mosquitoes are their airborne divisions. The swift and stealthy rat is their personnel carrier, stuffed with nimble fleas. The savage-clawed lice are their tenacious, mobile armoured vehicles of infection.

Our acquaintance Hieronymus Frascastorius of Verona first recognised typhus, 'spotted fever', sudden, prostrating, with a red rash and a 20 per cent death rate. American Howard Taylor Ricketts (1817–1910) found it was caused by one of the virus-like organisms which exist only inside living cells, which were named *Rickettsiae* after him – justly, because he died in Mexico City of typhus the year of his discovery. *Reckettsia prowazeki* is the specific organism causing typhus – and Stanislaus Josef Mathias von Prowazek (1875–1915) of Hamburg died of it, too. The microbes are sucked from infected man by the feeding louse, who jumps on to another human host and drops infected faeces on the skin, and the man does the rest by scratching. The poor louse turns red and dies, too.

> Ha! whare ye gaun, ye crowlin' ferlie!
> Your impudence protects you sairly:

Robert Burns wrote 'To a Louse', with his customary profound sympathy towards tiny creatures, with his gratitude for their example, and (to an Englishman) with his incomprehensibility.

What bring lice, bring typhus: war, human herding, dirt, no water nor fuel for washing, no clean shirt to change into. As 'gaol fever' in the sixteenth century, lice half-emptied the prisons and sportingly knocked off the judges by ascending to the bench at the assizes. At the Old Bailey in 1750, it executed three judges, the Lord Mayor of London, and eight of the jury. There must have been chortling in Newgate Gaol.

In 430 BC, typhus in Athens complicated the Peloponnesian War and killed Pericles (it may have been plague or smallpox, Thucydides' diagnosis is unreliable). At Antioch in 1098, typhus and dysentery did for the crusaders, man and horse. Widespread terror of infection elsewhere performed wonders for the Christian conversion-rate, particularly as the only public health measure was exorcism. During the Thirty Years War, the two sides squared up for the battle of Nürnberg in 1632, but typhus killed so many first that the fixture had to be scratched.

Typhus bedevilled King Charles' cavaliers at Oxford, and in 1741 captured Prague for Louis XV. With General Winter and its lieutenant dysentery, typhus accomplished the retreat from Moscow. (It was dysentery which raised the siege of Baghdad in 1439 and of Metz in 1553, and the victor of Agincourt died of the 'bloody flux' at Vincennes on 31 August 1422.) Lenin lost 3 million new comrades with typhus in 1918–22. It embellished the savageries of World War Two in concentration camps, refugee settlements and army depots, though the Allies beat the louse before the Nazis, extinguishing the Naples epidemic in 1944 by disinfection with DDT, an insecticide which now makes the Greens' hair stand up like rye-grass.

A typhus epidemic among the weavers of Upper Silesia in 1848 was investigated for the Prussians by Rudolf Virchow (1821–1902), from the Charité Hospital in Berlin.

33

His report so accurately condemned the local living and hygienic conditions, and so effectively indicated bountiful state aid as the only remedy, that the Prussians fired him. He got elected to the Reichstag, opposed Bismark, organised the Ambulance Corps of the Franco-Prussian war, and made the sewers of Berlin the envy of Europe.

This little, bouncy, snappy professor became a dominating European doctor, who first described leukaemia and was an expert on pulmonary embolism, lupus on the face, gout, tattooing and the archaeology of Troy. He struck the phrase: *Omnis cellula e cellula* – no disease creates its own cells, they are all the everyday cells of the human body, but distorted by disease. Nobody had thought of this before. When Jean Louis Armand de Quatrefages (1810–92) of the Natural History Museum in Paris wrote a pamphlet decrying the Prussians as a bunch of barbarian Mongols (they had just shelled his museum), Virchow furiously but solemnly recorded the hair colour and eye circularity of all 6 million German schoolchildren. His eightieth birthday was declared a national holiday, so the Prussians loved him in the end.

The Black Death

Now for the fleas.

Albert Camus in 1947 started *La Peste*, about Oran:

> When leaving his surgery on the morning of 16 April, Dr Bernard Rieux felt something soft under his foot. It was a dead rat lying in the middle of the landing. On the spur of the moment he kicked it to one side and, without giving it further thought, continued on his way downstairs. Only when he was stepping forth into the street did it occur to him that a dead rat had no business to be on his landing.

Coming home that evening, Dr Rieux encountered a tottering rat with blood spurting from its mouth, which gave a squeal and died. Next day, there were three dead rats in his hall. Soon, they were discovered in the Oran dustbins by the dozen. Then everywhere, in thousands. After a fortnight, 6,231 dead rats were burnt by the sanitary department in a day. Two days later, it was 8,000. People became disturbed.

As the rat flees the sinking ship, the flea quits the sinking rat. If the rat is dying from plague, then the short, fat, chain-forming *Pasteurella pestis* microbe, which is swarming in the blood of the flea's last meal, will be sicked up – yuk! – when the flea bites into its next one, often a man. Hence the Black Death of 1348.

The Black Death started on the shores of mountainous Lake Issyk-Kul, east of the Aral Sea, beyond Tashkent, in the corner between Russia and China north of the Himalayas. In 1346, the Black Death was killing Indians, Armenians, Tartars and Kurds, which did not over-bother anyone in Europe. Next year, it reached the Crimea, then Messina in Sicily, through rats aboard Genoese galleys. Next Genoa, Pisa and Venice. After that, there was no stopping it. At Christmas 1348 it was imported to England through Bristol, a year later it had swept the Highlands of Scotland. The doctors armoured themselves with long black leather gowns and gauntlets and prototypes of 1939 gas-masks, goggle-eyed with aromatic antiseptics in the snout. The patients burned herbs and sang psalms. The mortality among the conscientiously attending clergy was heroic.

It was the Black Death because the dead were black. They bled horribly into their skin. You could get two sorts: bubonic, with your lymph glands in your groins and armpits swollen like rotting oranges, the terrifying 'buboes'; or pneumonic, which was breathed from man to man, a bloody pneumonia, death certain and swift. Boccaccio's remark lingers:

> How many valiant men, how many fair ladies,
> breakfasted with their kinsfolk and that same night
> supped with their ancestors in the other world.

Into hastily dug pits were timorously shovelled the discoloured, putrefying, stinking, menacing corpses, in Europe twenty-five million of them, a quarter of its population. Half London perished, perhaps 50,000 people. Nobody knew what caused it, though the Jews were believed to be poisoning the wells.

Or was it so bad? In 1988, two emergency cemeteries dug in 1348 were excavated in London, near the Tower and in Smithfield. They were long sloping trenches, which had been sensibly filled deep end first, to save trundling dead over dead. The bodies were carefully arranged five deep and shallowly spread with earth, with separate graves for children. These burial-grounds indicate the City fathers' admirable foresight, when the plague was sweeping on them from the West country. The graves' 12,400 occupants – possibly most of London's casualties – indicate a tragedy less than traditional.

During the 1330s, Europe was already in economic recession, with trade languishing and prices falling, wars and riots disrupting commerce, harvests failing and food prices rocketing. Starvation struck, and the poor ate their dogs. At least, the Black Death solved the European overpopulation problem.

After the battle of Bosworth in 1485, the crowning of Henry VII was stopped by the sweating sickness. It was the only coronation postponed through illness until Edward VII's in the summer of 1901. *Sudor Anglicus* was a mysterious disease, the patients shivering and sweating and peculiarly stinking, and dying within the day. It was recorded by John Caius (1510–73), the physician who turned Gonville Hall at Cambridge into Gonville and Caius College, thereafter inflicting it with a preponderance of medical students. Caius was Court physician from Henry VIII to Elizabeth I, but a Reformation backslider. The Fellows of Caius nosed out his Catholic vestments and burnt them publicly, so he equally publicly put the Fellows in the stocks. His tomb in the College chapel says grumpily only: *Fui Caius*, I was Caius. He wrote also *Of English Dogges*.

The plague bells tolled again in London in 1563, when a fifth of its 93,000 population died, and in 1575, 1593, 1603, 1625 and 1636, each leaving 20,000 Londoners the fewer. The Black Death's most annotated sequel was the Great Plague of London.

In 1661 plague had returned to Turkey, in 1664 it killed a fifth of the population of Amsterdam and spread to Flanders, that December two Frenchmen died in Drury Lane, and the following June Samuel Pepys was recording:

> I did in Drury-lane see two or three houses marked
> with a red cross upon the doors, and 'Lord have mercy
> upon us' – which was a sad sight to me, being the first
> of that kind that to my remembrance I ever saw.

He bought some tobacco and chewed it to calm his nerves.

The regulation red cross was a foot high, the house was sealed and guarded for forty days, sick and well imprisoned together, food and medicine left warily on the doorstep. Their only visitors were brave doctors who had not fled London with the King, old women 'searchers' sent to discover from the fresh bodies' 'tokens' – crimson skin patches – what the victims had died of, and the nurses who robbed them and had sometimes impatiently strangled them, or had stealthily smeared their pus on the healthy to make another killing.

Nathaniel Hodges (1629–88), a jolly physician in trying circumstances, describes with satisfaction the nurse who waited until the whole family was killed, then dropped dead herself in the street outside, loaded with plunder. Another stripped her patient at his last gasp, but he recovered and 'came a second time into the world naked.'

Dr Hodges achieved immunity by sucking cinnamon lozenges while examing his patients, by eating plenty of roast meat and pickles ('indeed in this melancholy time the city greatly abounded with variety of all good things of that nature') and by a glass of sack before dinner, a few glasses with, and after his day's work 'drinking to cheerfulness of my old favourite liquor, which encouraged sleep and an easy breathing through the pores all night. Gratitude obliges me to do justice to the virtues of sack, as it is deservedly ranked among the principal antidotes.' He found the best sack was middle-aged – neat, fine, bright, racey and of a walnut flavour.

Nathaniel Hodges treated his patients with Virginian snake root, dried toad and doses of the College of Physicians' plague water, a pharmacological blunderbuss containing twenty-one remedies. When the plague was over he had no more patients, fell into poverty, was locked up in Ludgate Prison for debt, and died inside in 1688. An early example of the dangers in over-specialisation.

'Bring out your dead!' rang through the empty streets, and the bells tolled as the offerings were dumped by cartloads into pits. Dogs were suspected of passing the plague, and massacred. The rats got away with it. In the sultry September of 1665, when 12,000 Londoners were dying a week, the City fathers commanded fires to burn in the streets, three days on end, to purify the air. But the mourning heavens extinguished them. The physicians had disagreed with this idea as superfluous, showy and expensive. Exactly a year later, the Great Fire took exactly the same time to prove the physicians wrong.

Daniel Defoe's *Journal of the Plague Year*, published in 1722, was a skilful work of faction, like *Robinson Crusoe*.

The Shape of Plagues to Come

For another century bubonic plague killed lavishly in Malta, Vienna, Prague, Warsaw, and Copenhagen. In 1720 it culled almost half the population of Marseilles. In the 1930s it was still killing in Uganda, where cotton had been planted and its stored seed vastly increased the local rats.

Though plague petered out, there were four severe flu epidemics in Britain in the seventeenth century, ten in the eighteenth, six in the nineteenth, and in the twentieth the pandemic of 1918, which killed 0.5 per cent of the population of Britain and of the United States, and 25 million people throughout the world. The War just ended had killed 8,538,313 servicemen: so the flu virus slaughtered three times as many in a quarter of the time. Then this deadly sort of flu virus vanished. Perhaps it retreated into swine, from which it could return as alarmingly as did the vanquished of the Great War.

Nothing can cure flu. But antibiotics would today halt the fatal following pneumonia, as antibiotics can stop typhus, dysentery and plague. In our comfortable part of the world, where we are unthinkingly accustomed to cleanliness and clinicians, and where bacteriologists have now bettered themselves into 'microbiologists', viruses ravage mostly computers. We can feel smug plaguewise

Can we?

In 1967 this world was startled by a new disease. It

was borne by green monkeys destined for the experimental benches of a research institute at Marburg in Western Germany. Seven humans died, among the laboratory staff and among the doctors and nurses attending them. The monkeys carried an unknown virus from central Africa, somewhere north of Lake Victoria, probably originating in the funnel-webbed spider, an insect clearly to be avoided. From this area – where regrettably sex is not performed exclusively on Slumberland mattresses behind Laura Ashley curtains after the television finishes – came the AIDS virus. There is no cure for either of these imported diseases. Nor will there be cures for another, and another, and yet another, mysteriously appearing and giving us something deadly else . . .

H. G. Wells, comfortable in the time machine a century later, is busy on the Martians' sequel.

There are some kindly bacteria. They help the growth of pulses, which men eat, and of clover, which cows eat. Without bacteria, we should never enjoy garden peas, butter beans and Sunday's roast beef.

THREE

Discoveries in the Dark

Great medical breakthroughs were accomplished without the slightest idea of what was being broken through.

The Doctor and the Milkmaid

Attend to Thomas Hardy:

> The season developed and matured. Dairyman Crick's
> household of maids and men lived on comfortably,
> placidly, even merrily. Their position was perhaps the
> happiest of all positions in the social scale, beginning
> above the line at which neediness ends, and below the
> line at which *convenances* begin to cramp natural
> feeling, and the stress of threadbare modishness makes
> too little of enough.
> Milking was done betimes; and before the milking

came the skimming, which began at a little past three. There was a great stir in the milk-house just after breakfast. The churn revolved as usual, but the butter would not come. Whenever this happened the dairy was paralysed. Squish, squash echoed the milk in the great cylinder, but never arose the sound they waited for.

A figure came unexpectedly past the door. Curious, the maiden left the singular, luminous gloom, for the light which pervaded the open mead. There stood a handsome gentleman in buckskins and top-boots with silver spurs, some forty-five years of age, of fresh face, thick fair hair, a kindly mouth and cordial yet quizzical blue eye. Her own teeth, lips, and eyes scintillated in the sunbeams, she was again the dazzlingly fair dairymaid, who had to hold her own against the other women of the world.

'Well, my beauty, what can I do for you?' said he. She curtsied. 'And what do they call you?'

'Tess, sir.'

'You are blessed that so fair a face has escaped the savage bite of the prowling spotted beast, the smallpox,' he said, with a pleased gleam in his face.

'But I can't take smallpox, sir, because I have already had cowpox.'

The gentleman crashed fist into palm, and cried, as loud as a startled swan: 'By God! I've got it!'

She almost jumped out of her pattens.

So one of England's most significant novelists (and one of its most insignificant) describe Edward Jenner's (1749–1823) discovery of vaccination.

The Benevolent Udder

The complexions of English milkmaids had been admired in poem and song since the sixteenth century. In the eighteenth century, the milkmaids of Gloucestershire were regularly discovering – with greater resignation than annoyance, and never with alarm – spots on their arms, and on the hands which early every morning tweaked the teats. They caught such blemishes from the sores of cowpox, a common udder infection in dairy herds. After a week, the spots turned into pustules, and the milkmaids suffered a passing illness like the influenza. But once the sticky blebs had scabbed and flaked, there endured with the scars the comfort of celebrated immunity to smallpox. And the only milkmaids who never caught cowpox were those who had luckily recovered from smallpox.

This immunological curiosity had been known throughout the shires for years – the squires with their crystal-borne brandy, the yeoman puffing their church-wardens, doubtless discussed it endlessly round winter's fires. Why, down in Dorset in 1774, farmer Benjamin Jesty had enterprisingly given his wife and sons the protective cowpox disease, with a cobbler's needle transferring pus straight from the sore udder. Dr Fewster had even brought the rustic coincidence to the notice of the London Medical Society in 1765, but nobody took any notice.

On Saturday, 14 May 1796, Dr Jenner from Berkeley, a village by the River Severn between Gloucester and the prosperous slave-trading port of Bristol, took a gob of pus from cowpox-infected Sara Nelmes, a farmer's daughter, and with two light half-inch scratches implanted it into the arm of eight-year old James Phipps. Sarah had three isolated open pustules, an inch across, on the forefinger, ball of thumb and wrist of her right hand. They were bluish with raised edges, and she had swollen glands in her armpit. Sara had just been badly infected on the hand by the scratch of a thorn, like Florey's first penicillin patient 145 years later.

Jenner had pondered this transference idea for twenty

years before putting it into possibly perilous practice. He had become the club bore about it at the local Convivio-Medical, the members groaning over their claret to chuck him out – as Alexander Fleming, 130 years later, bored the Research Club in London about his bacteria-dissolving mould juice. The difference was, Jenner enjoyed the imagination to put his notion into clinical practice, and Fleming did not.

On 1 July, Jenner scratched the lad James with human smallpox pus. Nothing happened. He repeated this dose of human pus after some months. Still nothing happened. He had invented *vaccination* (a *vacca* browsed and mooed on ancient Roman fields). But Jenner was not taking the heartless, undue, or unknown risk that his failure would be indicated by the child's death from induced smallpox. *Inoculation* with human smallpox pus, not cows' cowpox pus, had been around for longer than beautiful milkmaids.

The ancient Chinese perhaps inoculated against smallpox by sniffing a snuff of its pus. The Turks had certainly been inoculating for generations. They gave small parties, attended by old women who needled smallpox venom into their skins from a nutshell. These social functions excited the wife of the British ambassador to Constantinople, Lady Mary Wortley Montague (1689–1762). She had recovered from smallpox aged twenty-six, disfigured for life.

> Now beauty's fled, and lovers are no more . . .
> Could no pomatum save a trembling maid?

she sighed in a pathetic poem.

Her younger brother had died of smallpox. Her six-year-old son she determinedly had inoculated against it, on 18 March 1718. Lady Montague eagerly imported the Turkish technique into England, where it was offered as

Hobson's choice to six London criminals awaiting execution. It proved a startlingly successful alternative to the gallows. The doctors were as delighted as the hangmen disappointed. Though one condemned man kept mum that he had already recovered from smallpox, and so was immune anyway. And as a clinical control, another criminal was given the legendary Chinese treatment of dried pustules up the nostrils, developed mild smallpox, recovered, and was spared the rope. She was a girl of eighteen.

Several Royals took confidence from so dutiful an example by their wayward subjects, and got inoculated, too. Soon, everyone was doing it. The doctors nicked the arm, and pulled through a thread heavy with somebody's smallpox pus. Which, with good luck, provoked mild smallpox and lifelong immunity. With bad, it gave you full-blown smallpox and killed you. The Church meanwhile objected that it took the power out of God's hand.

The Spotted Menace

The eighteenth was the century of smallpox terror. The late seventeenth had suffered epidemics in England and New England, and by slaying Red Indians wholesale it had assisted the palefaces to inherit America. It ravaged families: diarist John Evelyn in 1685 lost his daughters Mary in March and Elizabeth in August. Apprentices and smart lads seeking hire were demanded to have had smallpox, to save catching it and killing off their masters; maidservants advertised their recovery from it as proudly as their sobriety. Fairs and markets were ruinously cancelled by it, pubs advertised that they were well aired and free from it, it claimed one in five deaths and almost everybody got it. In 1746, 3,236 Londoners died in the smallpox epidemic, the victims were buried in terror at night, farm cart for hearse, the bearers buoyed with beer, the tolling bell falling silent as the clerk sobered up and fled. Though the pockmarks were useful for identifying runaway husbands and criminals, and in 1739 did for Dick Turpin.

London soon sprouted fashionable inoculators like Quaker Thomas Dimsdale (1712–1800), who was summoned in 1768 to inoculate Catharine the Great of Russia and her son the Grand Duke Paul. The idea was Voltaire's. It is difficult to philosophise whether it scotched, or fortified, his notion that doctors pour drugs of which they know little, to cure diseases of which they know less, into human beings of which they know nothing. Dimsdale got £10,000 down, £2,000 expenses, £500 pension and a Russian barony. High stakes, but the patients would not have been the only fatalities had things gone wrong (Dimsdale had prudently laid his escape route). He inoculated 200 Russians, his first child patient graciously commanded by the Empress to be rechristened 'Vaccinoff', poor dear.

Robert Sutton (?1708–88) and his son Daniel inoculated more prudently by puncture, not incision, and advertised commodious inoculation houses round London for suffering the inevitable mild attack, with full board of fish, fowl and mutton (wine, but not tea and sugar, included) at two guineas a week. They had 30,000 patients with a trivial 4 per cent mortality, and made fortunes despite the envy of rival inoculators, the ire of the Royal College of Physicians (Daniel was inconveniently unqualified) and the outrage of their houses' neighbours.

Inoculators were curious about an oddity in their practice: it never worked if the patient had suffered cowpox. Jenner milked the answer. Sarah was his case No 16 of cowpox. From the others, seen over twenty-five years, he formalised the Gloucestershire legend:

- Cowpox patients never caught smallpox in its epidemics.
- Milkmaids who had recovered from smallpox never got cowpox.
- But cowpox sufferers could get cowpox again, two or three times.
- And milkmaids could give their cowpox to cows.

Vaccination speedily ousted inoculation as safer – because you could not develop smallpox from it – and socially preferable, because the cowpox sufferer could not spread smallpox, and the inoculated mild smallpox sufferer could. In 1840 inoculation became a felony.

A Country Gentleman

Edward Jenner was the son of the vicar of Berkeley, his mother the daughter of the vicar before. At thirteen, he was apprenticed to a surgeon at Chipping Sodbury, but he grew into more than the risky rural GP. At St George's Hospital at Hyde Park Corner he was a prized pupil of John Hunter (1728–93), the man who turned surgery from barbering into science. Hunter was an anatomist of creatures great and small, he dissected them from bees to whales. The 13,600 specimens cramming his museum in Leicester Square included the famed skeleton of Irish giant Mr Byrne, which Hunter fancied during life and bought for £500, after use (Sir Joshua Reynolds got the picture). Hunter was a scornful and proud Scotsman, a dreadful lecturer, who, the students said, had a skeleton once brought in that he might begin: 'Gentlemen – ' He had syphilis, which he gave himself by inoculation to prove it was different from gonorrhea (his story). And angina, of which he kept reflecting: 'My life is in the hands of any rascal who chooses to annoy and tease me,' until one so did, at a meeting of the St George's governors. John Hunter was buried at St Martin's-in-the-Fields, but was dug up in 1859 in favour of Westminster Abbey, the Royal College of Surgeons paying for the removal.

'Why think? Why not try the experiment?' Hunter was continually urging – an aphorism which, with Jenner, clearly if belatedly sank in. The pair became lifelong friends. Hunter wrote to him in Berkeley in 1778, after Jenner was jilted:

> I own I was glad when I heard you was married to a woman of fortune. But let her go, never mind her. I shall employ you with hedgehogs. I want you to get a hedgehog in the beginning of winter, and weigh him; put him in your garden, and let him have some leaves, hay, or straw to cover himself with, then weigh him in the spring and see what he has lost. I want you to kill one in the beginning of winter, to see how fat he is, and another in the spring, to see what he has lost of his fat.

Nothing like the needles of hedgehogs for sewing a broken heart. (The lady is a mystery, though Eleanor Clutterbuck and Judith Excell of Wooton-under-Edge flit into medical history as desirable local heiresses at the time.) Jenner played the flute and wrote poetry – 'Address to a Robin' and 'Signs of Rain':

> The hollow winds begin to blow,
> The clouds look black, the glass is low,
> The soot falls down, the spaniels sleep,
> And spiders from their cobwebs creep,

and so on.

He was a kindly medical squire, deserving the ready touch of a forelock. He later built a cottage for his experimental James Phipps, himself planting the roses in the garden. In his own garden, Jenner turned a thatched stone hut, installed to impart a sylvan look, into the Temple of Vaccina where he did the poor free. By then, he was tranisferring person-to-person, the cow had quickly become redundant.

Stop Vaccination Now!

Like any fresh ideas blowing through any establishment, Jenner's found the windows quickly shut. The Royal Society rejected them snootily:

> He ought not to risk his reputation by presenting to the learned body anything which appeared so much at variance with established knowledge, and withal so incredible.

Perhaps they jibbed at the full thirty-three-word title of An Enquiry into the Causes and Effects etc ... his slim, elegantly written volume presenting the heresy with coloured illustrations of elegant milkmaids' hands, 7s 6d.

People worried about being converted into cows:

> There, nibbling at thistle, stand Jem, Joe, and Mary,
> On their foreheads, O horrible! crumpled horns bud;
> There Tom with his tail, and poor William all hairy,
> Reclined in a corner, are chewing the cud,

went the comic song.

But vaccination caught on. In 1800, 6,000 enjoyed the milkmaid's bounty. In 1802 Parliament voted Jenner £10,000, in 1807 another £20,000, historical generosity with the taxpayers' money. He became a Freeman of London and MD of Oxford, and was created a Fellow of the red-faced Royal Society. When Napoleon was implored by Jenner in 1813 to release a captured relative, the Emperor exclaimed: 'Ah! C'est Jenner, je ne puis rien refuser à Jenner.' Jenner's response to all this was: 'And what is Fame? A gilded butt, for ever pierced with the arrows of malignancy', which must often have occurred to anybody who ever got into the papers.

People continued to die of smallpox. Only the nobs could afford vaccination. The remedy was free vaccination for all infants, which was provided in Britain in 1840 and made compulsory in 1853 (after Bavaria, Denmark, Sweden, Würtemberg and Prussia). But for any activity whatever in Britain, a society is always founded to stop it. Today, the Scotch Whisky Association in Edinburgh toasts the National Temperance League in Sheffield, the Masters of Foxhounds cry 'Tally-ho!' across the Cotswolds at the League Against Cruel Sports in the Elephant and Castle, the Naval and Military Club in Piccadilly sights over its port the teacups of the International Friendship League in Acton, even the Royal College of Surgeons in Lincoln's Inn Fields must acknowledge the Patients Association down in the East End. So Jenner's spirit in 1867 faced the Anti-Vaccination League.

> The cutting with a sharp instrument of holes in your dear little healthy babe's arm, a few weeks after it is born, and putting into the holes some filthy matter from a cow . . .

said the League.

Enough to make a crocodile weep.

The League staged a big demo in 1885, the future prime minister Balfour intervened, vaccination became a political drama, and like all political drama, up to the running of our ramshackle National Health Service, the script was henceforth written by Lewis Carroll. The Antis even achieved the stopping of compulsory vaccination in the Forces in the year of the Battle of the Somme.

By 1899, parents were allowed to entertain conscientious objection against vaccination, towards which the public attitude settled into apathy enlivened by panic during any local epidemic. But mass vaccination won. In World War Two, England had only three smallpox deaths. Jenner's triumph was proclaimed paradoxically in 1946, when our Ministry of Health awoke to the danger of infrequent deaths from vaccination now outweighing the danger of even rarer deaths from smallpox. So in 1948, compulsory vaccination of infants was stopped, though voluntary vaccination continued free, to express the bounties of the new National Health Service.

In 1971, routine voluntary vaccination of infants was abolished. In 1977 smallpox was eradicated from the world. How pleasant to end with such gratifying simplicity.

Something in the Air

Jenner had worked out, anticipating Louis Pasteur:

> The source of smallpox is morbid matter of a peculiar kind.

And Jenner had speculated, anticipating Robert Koch:

> May we not conceive that many contagious diseases, now prevalent among us, may owe their present appearance not to a simple, but to a compound origin? For example, it is difficult to imagine that the measles, the scarlet fever, and the ulcerous sore throat with a

spotted skin, have all sprung from the same source, assuming some variety in their forms according to the nature of their new combinations?

Jenner had no more idea than the cow that smallpox was caused by a virus. Under an electron microscope, this virus is shaped like a brick, a big one of the deoxyribonucleic acid group. It grows on chick embryos, and gives them visible smallpox in three days. The cowpox virus is much the same, though the world's vaccinators kissed the milkmaids goodbye, and performed with the smallpox virus attenuated by passing it through calves.

A century ago, when new microbes were being identified annually, doctors remained dreadfully muddled about germs. The notion of infection did not dawn upon them as a glorious sunrise deserving scientific contemplation. That outburst of discovery detonated by Robert Koch in 1876 was so violent, that instead of gently illuminating the ancient architecture of medical thought it reduced it to ruins.

Even Hieronymus Fracastorius' ancient 'fomites' were invoked to explain these mysterious new 'contagium particles', which Dr Husband of Edinburgh was vaguely instructing students fifteen years after Koch: 'Are said to possess an independent life, capable of moving about in fluids, searching for food, growing and dying.'

Some conflicting professional opinions:

- Dr Parkes explained that infection was not inevitable, because some persons did not embody these particles' proper food, or it had been all eaten up by them in an earlier attack.
- Professor Hallier decided the particles were fungi.
- Dr Ross quoted Darwin to insist that contagium particles were modified bits of an individual which

became detached, and produced disease by grafting themselves on to somebody else.

— Dr Richardson thought they released undue oxygen from the blood, decomposing the tissues.

— The Medical Officer of the Privy Council calculated officially: 'A single bacterium will produce 16,777,220 individuals every twenty-four hours.'

Infection then was an affliction of largely impotent argument, like cancer now.

But disinfectants like Dr Condy's fluid were already being splashed about lavishly at the middle of the century, and deodorants appeared in public health textbooks long before they reached sophisticated armpits. Eau-de-Cologne was the favourite perfume for disguising the disgusting gangrenous hospital stinks. Mysterious 'fermentations' and 'putrefactions' had to be prevented from producing their nebulous 'contagia': so carbolic acid, potassium permanganate and chlorine came to be used, rightly and effectively, to prevent infection by the germs of which everyone was ignorant (Hippocrates had used tar).

Direct contact of disinfectant and contagium was, also correctly, seen as essential; the mere air of the sickroom reeking with carbolic was justly condemned as futile. Dry heat to 125° C was advised as the most efficient disinfectant of all, the perceptive precursor of modern sterilisation. 'It is to cleanliness, ventilation, and drainage,' the Privy Council Medical Officer was admirably directing, back in 1866, 'and the use of perfectly pure drinking water, that populations ought mainly to look for safety against nuisance and infection.' Miss Nightingale had sternly foreseen as much in Scutari. To Miss Nightingale, cleanliness was all. Miss Nightingale throughout a long life regarded germs as slightingly as male supremacy.

Though the enemy was still unknown, the incitement to kill it was 'hospitalism': the infection, blood-poisoning and green-black gangrene which emptied surgical wards into the graveyard, and awarded successive occupants of the operating table a worse chance than a guardsman at Waterloo.

Joseph Lister (1827–1912), a London wine-merchant's son, was a student spectator of Robert Liston's performing the first European operation under anaesthesia at University College Hospital in 1846. Lister studied inflammation in frogs' feet. He speculated that the fatal infection of surgical wounds was imparted not by the popular, vague notion of miasmas, but by something solid floating in the air. Like Jenner, Lister anticipated Louis Pasteur, who in 1864 elucidated these invisible particles as living things, which acidified wine. It flashed upon Joseph Lister that, if solid things putrefied the wine which his father sold, they might equally putrefy the wounds which he himself created.

Lister ingeniously sought to destroy this mass of still wholly unsorted germs where the surgeon's knife admitted them, by swamping the operation area with a disinfectant. He chose carbolic acid, which he knew worked a treat on the sewage of Carlisle. Lister was then Professor of Surgery at Glasgow Royal Infirmary, which was built on a graveyard crammed from the cholera epidemics. He tried out his idea on 12 August 1865, applying lint soaked in carbolic to the left leg of eleven-year old Jimmy Greenlees, who had a fractured tibia poking through the skin.

Lister next adapted the spray which ladies' dressing-tables provided for scent, with a student dresser turning its handle on a tasselled occasional table as used for afternoon tea. The surgical team wore the same clothes they had arrived in, though in a workmanlike way the operator turned back his cuffs. Some surgeons preserved their socially worn-out frock-coats for operating, their thread ligatures dangling handily in the buttonhole, stiff with blood and pus, the filthier the coat proclaiming the busier their practice. The operating theatre had kitchen sinks with brass taps, marble-topped bathroom tables for the bottles and towels, china basins holding the gory sponges, and a pail of sand with a coal-shovel to overlay the sticky blood on the floorboards. A coke stove warmed in winter, and facilitated the more conservative surgeons' stanching the bleeding with red-hot irons, as did their Elizabethan ancestors.

Lister's scent-spray was bettered by his 'donkey engine', a wooden tripod supporting a jar of carbolic acid vaporised by a levered hand-pump (viewable in the hallway of the Royal College of Surgeons). Inevitably, it was soon worked by steam like the railways and the liners. The discomfort for the surgical team of a pungent phenol cloud in their faces, day after day, will be appreciated by any dutiful gardener who in breezy January ventures to spray his fruit trees. In 1887, Lister dropped the donkey engine, reverting to gauze impregnated with carbolic.

In 1871, Lister operated on the royal armpit. Queen Victoria suffered an abscess six inches across in her left axilla, which was worse than painful, it was considered undignified. In the awesome atmosphere of the operation, performed under local, the Queen unfortunately got a blast of the spray full in the face. 'I am only the man who works the bellows,' miserably protested the assistant catching the regal wrath. Lister boasted delicately after Victoria's death: 'I believe that I happen to be the only person who ever exercised upon her sacred body the divine art of surgery.' Among friends, he put it: 'Gentlemen, I am the only man who has ever stuck a knife into the Queen!'

On his seventieth birthday Lister met Pasteur arriving on the arm of President Carnot at the Sorbonne. 'There does not exist in the wide world an individual to whom medical science owes more than to you,' said Lister to Pasteur graciously. They kissed, and everyone shouted 'Vive!' At this academic back-scratching, Lister had been a lord for three months, medicine's first.

Cleaning Up

Lister's ideas did not make a clean sweep of his profession. In the 1880s, the less muddled London surgeons would grudgingly admit the existence of bacteria, but jibbed at the notion of their creating disease under their own fingertips. A knighted physician at King's College Hospital, who idly poked an inquiring forefinger into Lister's incision, found himself flung violently from the operating-table by the surgeon. Sanitation in an operating theatre was widely derided as finical, ladylike and affected, the equivalent of the block being scrubbed before use by a butcher or a headsman.

Robert Lawson Tait (1845–99) was a gynaecologist in burgeoning Birmingham who fiercely absolved bacteria from causing the 'laudable pus' which dripped so freely from surgical wounds. But he was exceptional in lavishing soap and hot water on his operating theatre with the zeal of a houseproud wife, and his ovariotomies lived. Eugène Koeberlé (1828–1915) in Alsace did his ovariotomies after flaming his instruments, and Ernst von Bergmann (1836–1907) in Berlin sterilised everything by steam. The idea that cleanliness was next to the surgeon's familiar godliness was catching on.

Lister's *antiseptic* method of killing germs on operating fields was replaced everywhere towards the end of his life by *asepsis*, using autoclaves and boiling water to prevent their appearance in the first place. Only fifteen years after Jimmy Greenlees' operation in Glasgow, William Stewart Halstead (1852–1922) at Johns Hopkins Hospital in Baltimore was performing not antiseptic but aseptic surgery. Surgical gowns were preboiled, and surgical rubber gloves were donned in 1890, following Professor Halstead's distress that Miss Hampton, his scrub nurse, was staining her sensitive hands. The experiment was so successful that the Professor married her the same year. Lister meanwhile fought against the new idea, as bitterly as the horse-breeder against the motorcar, the cavalry colonel against the tank, and his own stubborn opponents of the donkey-engine.

Nowadays asepsis is all, the instruments are sterilised remotely by gamma rays and delivered in handy paper packets like Band-aid, the surgeons are attired in the sterile gowns, caps, masks and gloves which have become, to a devoted TV world audience, traditional ceremonial drapings like the copes and chasubles of the Church.

The division of surgical history into pre- and post-Listerian epochs still venerates Lister for opening up the body's holy places – the joints, the abdomen, the chest, the skull – previously sealed by the devils of infection. But the identification and acceptance of germs towards the end of the nineteenth century would anyway have achieved this, even had Lister followed his father into the wine trade.

'Let us hear no more of the nonsense about the bad results in surgery of pre-Listerian times as having been cured by Lister. It is not the truth,' Lawson Tait wrote in an ungentlemanly way in 1898. Perhaps the cad was right. Shots in the dark are rendered unnecessary by patiently waiting for daybreak. Yet: 'No one knew how to render a pin-prick harmless or dress a finger till Lister came!'

Hard Tack

All stood together on the deck,
For a charnel-dungeon fitter:
All fix'd on me their stony eyes,
That in the Moon did glitter.

Samuel Taylor Coleridge,
The Rime of the Ancient Mariner.

Swollen, spongy, purplish, bleeding gums, filthy breath, teeth loose then spat out, spotty bleeding round the body hairs, soon huge bruises, swollen joints, bloody nose, bloody eyes, bloody vomit, unhealed wounds, lassitude, feebleness, heart failure and sudden death. When the hardy seafarers ventured from Bristol in the eighteenth century, leaving Dr Jenner among the milkmaids, all this was as common afloat as seasickness.

Vasco de Gama, in 1497 first round the Cape of Good Hope, had lost 100 of 160 crew from it. The disease had mystified Ferdinand Magellan, the first to navigate Cape Horn in 1520: a year and a quarter out of Seville, three months from overwintering at San Julian in Patagonia, his men's 'gums grew so over their teeth that they died miserably for hunger.' Jacques Cartier from St Malo, discoverer of the St Lawrence, spending the winter of 1535 at anchor in the St Charles river that divides Quebec, lost fifty men in December when this 'unknown sickness began to spread itself amongst us in the strangest sort that ever was either heard of or seen.' By February, he had barely ten fit hands of 110, another twenty-five died ashore in March, despite continual prayer.

Armada veteran Sir Richard Hawkins, author of *Voyage into the South Sea*, followed Drake's wake to circumnavigate the globe in *Repentance* (renamed by order of Queen Elizabeth I *Daintie*), bountifully provisioned in 1593 at

Plymouth with beef, pork, biscuit and cider, and encountered the affliction on the Equator. In his twenty years at sea, Sir Richard reckoned to have seen 10,000 cases of it.

Scurvy was a disease to be piloted by dead reckoning. Commanders puzzled whether it were an infection by mysterious fomites, or caused by the obvious laziness of its sufferers, by unwholesome miasmas 'tween-decks, the salt in the air, the hard life, kissing women ashore, the victuals. The Navy's daily ration in 1615 was eight ounces of cheese, four ounces of bacon and four of butter, and a pound of biscuit, often wormy and 'stinking like pisse', but tolerable with the gallon of beer.

Sea scurvy was severe and swift, rare in officers, even petty officers, striking quicker if the voyage started in spring. On the convict hulks moored off Woolwich in the Thames, scurvy played the busy hangman. The slave traders fretted aboard their crammed vessels that it was ruinously costing them valuable lives. Land scurvy more insidiously attacked garrisons, the besieged, the Low Countries, the north of Russia and Scandinavia, and the Roman legions got it once they had crossed the Rhine.

Luckily for the Romans, the Dutch had a curative herb, and so did the Indians bordering the St Lawrence. Amazed at a dying Indian who recovered in a week by drinking a tea of sprouting pine-needles, Jacques Cartier enthusiastically brewed up for his crew and watched them mend, his gratification the warmer for having just opened a dead friend in the snow without finding reason for the engorged scorbutic body.

Lemons and Limes

The age believed that for every ill which God wrathfully inflicted he mercifully planted a herb to cure it. The herbal echoed the Bible.

James I's herbalist and barber-surgeon John Gerarde (1545–1612) in 1597 divinely proclaimed scurvy grass. This foot-high, white-flowered *Cochlearia officinalis*, flourishing beside the sea, is one of the four-petalled cruciferae family, related to turnips, radishes, watercress, mustard and wallflowers. The street-cry 'Buy any scurvy-grass!' was well enough known to be used in Middleton and Decker's *The Roaring Girl* of 1611. By 1661, you could buy scurvy-grass ale. In 1764, Byron's grandfather Admiral 'Foul-weather Jack' prudently provisioned *Dolphin* for a voyage round the world with scurvy-grass and coconuts.

Sailors were discovering that tropical fruit eaten ashore cured scurvy aboard. Sour oranges and lemons were Sir Richard Hawkins' favourite ration, and the East India Company's surgeon John Woodall (1569–1643) in *The Surgeon's Mate* of 1612 recommended lemon-juice to be stored aboard all the Company's ships. The Dutch preferred *Sauerkraut*, and Captain Cook swore by carrot marmalade and brewers' wort. Vinegar, swallowed or for swabbing the decks, oil of vitriol, and burial of the patient up to the neck in cold earth, all had their champions, if misguided.

James Lind (1716–94) of Edinburgh, nine years at sea with the Navy, bravely outspoken against the sickly accommodation, the rancid food, the foul water, came ashore as physician to the Haslar Naval Hospital in Portsmouth, which in 1790 still housed 1,754 cases of scurvy. Scurvy had lost Lord Anson three-quarters of his crew who rounded the world in 1740–44; in 1778 the Channel Fleet after ten weeks at sea had 2,400 cases. But in 1753 Lind's *Treatise of the Scurvy* had set a course through the flotsam of causes and cures still floating on a sea of ignorance.

On 20 May 1747, aboard *Salisbury*, homeward bound a month out of Plymouth, Lind conducted a clinical trial.

Twelve scurvy patients lay in the forepeak sick-bay, eating gruel for breakfast, mutton-broth and pudding for dinner, sago with currants and raisins for supper. Lind gave two of them a quart of cider a day. Two had oil of vitriol. Two vinegar. Two sea-water. Two had oranges and lemons, and two a pet electuary of garlic, radish, Peru balsam and myrrh. The pair on oranges and lemons were fit for duty in six days, and put to nurse the others who remained persistently sick.

Johannes Bachstrom (1686–1742) of Leyden had thirteen years earlier declared sea and land scurvy one disease with one cure: eating up your greens. Lind protested similarly that:

> The ignorant sailor and the learned physician will
> equally long, with the most craving anxiety, for green
> vegetables and the fresh fruits of the earth.

Lind prescribed lemon or lime juice.

He had found the specific remedy, with no notion how it worked, to a disease for which nobody remotely knew the reason.

The year after his death the Admiralty agreed with him. An ounce of lemon juice with an ounce and a half of sugar was issued to all hands after six weeks at sea. Scurvy vanished like the Flying Dutchman.

The lemon juice was later agreeably preserved by adding a quarter of its volume of rum. Masters of merchant ships were forced from 1854: 'To serve out the lime or lemon juice to the crew whenever they have consumed salt provisions for ten days'. West Indian limes were commercially favourable to Mediterranean lemons, and christened us enduringly on the American seaboard (though Limeys for a while were also the 'new chums' off the boat in Australia). Limes were puzzlingly not as effective against scurvy as lemons. Sir George Nares' search for the North Pole on lime-juice in 1875 was scorbutic, Sir Alexander Armstrong's on lemons in 1850 was not. Sometimes 85 per cent of Miss Nightingale's patients at Scutari had scurvy despite the ration of lime-juice, but this was readily explained by all of it lying forgotten at Balaclava. The right answer had to wait fifty years.

The Spice of Life

Vitamins are chemicals in food clinically conspicuous by their absence. They were invented in Cambridge in 1912 by Sir Frederick Gowland Hopkins (1861–1947). Ageing Cantabrigian doctors like myself can remember his inspiring the hushed 'It's Hopkins!' – like Pasteur or Lister – when he manifested in the Biochemistry Labs between Pembroke and Downing Colleges.

Hopkins discovered that one minute drop of milk could render impeccable a diet which was killing rats. He was also the posthumous father-in-law of J. B. 'Good Companions' Priestley.

In 1907, scurvy was given to guinea-pigs in Norway. It was then sinking into nutritional scientists that man's food may chemically consist exclusively of protein, fat, carbohydrate, and minerals, but some additive was mysteriously necessary. Those mice of Hopkins had flourished on milk alone. But fed on milk's separated constituents, they died.

In 1932, vitamin C was crystallised by mistake by Szent Györgi in Hungary, then in America from lemon-juice as ascorbic acid. It was a simple chemical which cured scurvy and sorted its confusions: lemons were more effective than limes because three times richer in vitamin C, the better-fed officers left port with more vitamin C aboard their bodies, in spring the whole crew sailed at their winter lowest from scant vegetables. Vitamin C is made internally by all animals, except for those experimental guinea-pigs, us, and monkeys.

In 1886, the Dutch had been worried about beri-beri in the East Indies. Beri-beri means in Singhalee 'I cannot', indicating the helplessness of its wasted muscles or swollen legs, preceding death from heart failure. Dutch army doctor Christiaan Eijkman (1858–1930) thought beri-beri an infection, until underfunding in 1897 obliged him to feed his experimental chickens on hospital leftovers, and they got it. If the white polished rice of curries and puddings was replaced by unappetising greyish unpolished rice, they got better. He tried polished rice on the chickens with replacement fat and minerals. No good. He tried polished rice and a meagre extract of the rice polishings, and the chickens were soon busily scratching and laying. Eijkman declared in 1901 that the recognised items of diet needed an unknown 'something else', in minuscule amounts, and of no nutritional value, to keep us alive. But nobody took much notice. His something was the vitamin B in the rice germ attached to the polished away skin. This was apparent only after Hopkins had applied his imagination to the puzzle. All ended happily, in 1929 they shared the Nobel Prize.

The other vitamins were steadily identified and synthesised before 1940. Vitamin A in milk, butter, eggs and fish liver oils prevents forms of blindness. B is several vitamins from cereals, which prevent various skin disorders, pellagra (dermatitis, diarrhoea and dementia), and the beri-beri suffered by Eijkman's chickens and also by 40 per cent of the Japanese navy between 1878–82. D, which comes with A, prevents rickets; K in green vegetables prevents undue bleeding. Nobody knows what vitamin E does. When discovered in 1936 it was believed to increase fertility, causing those ageing Cambridge doctors to sing topically:

Vitamin E is the thing for me!
We'll dash the hopes of Marie Stopes
By taking it in our tea.

In our well-housed, healthy and hedonistic world,
vitamin deficiency is suffered only by the decrepit who
cannot eat a normal diet and the faddists who will not.
What made miserable dietetic history for us all now
occurs predominately in the comparatively newly discovered Third World. This is a land of which we are
vaguely aware, consisting of forests where it is always
raining and nothing grows, where there is little to do but
copulation, where the natives wear tattered tartan
dinner-jackets and kipper ties while watching black-and-
white TV and listening to vinyl records in their huts,
sitting on plastic chairs and lying on futons, amid a
profusion of other items we have for years gratefully got
rid of to Oxfam. Vitamin A-deficient keratomalacia alone
blinds a hundred thousand children there every year, but
nobody does much about it.

Vitamin C does not cure colds, heal wounds nor sober
you up. Vitamin A does not make you see in the dark
(RAF disinformation in 1940, it was really radar). An
overdose of vitamin A or D can make you ill, but no
vitamins can make you healthier. They cannot increase
your children's intelligence. As they are not free on the
NHS, they are an unintelligent waste of money. A recent
British Prime Minister took a tablet of vitamin C every
morning.

The Foxglove

'If Winter comes, can Spring be far behind?' was a damn
stupid remark of Shelley's, though admittedly he was
living in Italy at the time. When winter comes to

England, spring is still beyond the next Grand National and sometimes well into the cricket season. But once English woods wear a green blush and night starts lifting her skirts, we celebrate our escape from the medical perils of winter by enjoying the offerings of the ripening earth – like strawberries, asparagus, and new potatoes, now all so conveniently flown in from California, Chile and Egypt.

When Shakespeare was talking about 'the green lap of the new come spring,' we cleansed the winter blood in a homely way by taking tea made from the new come herbs: yellow ox-eye (like marigolds), the water-weed Hampshire purslane, or from raspberry leaves or last season's blackcurrant jam, or from turnip juice (you extract it by sugaring raw slices). These teas were unbeknown antiscorbutics, like Lind's lime-juice, admirable when the vitamin C in equinoctial blood was running low.

William Withering (1741–99) was a rural GP in Stafford making £100 a year, who moved to Birmingham and made £1,000 a year, but loved getting out into the country. Birmingham had been a busy manufacturing town since armouring Cromwell with 15,000 sword blades for the Civil War. It attracted practical chaps, like Joseph Priestley who discovered oxygen, James Watt who invented railways, William Herschel who discovered Uranus, John Smeaton who made the Eddystone lighthouse, and Josiah Wedgwood who made the plates. They turned themselves into the Lunar Society, to discuss science and philosophy every full moon. Withering was their botanist. His *A Botanical Arrangement of all Vegetables Naturally Growing in Great Britain* was the enormous success of 1776. He was chief physician to the Birmingham General Hospital, combining the expertise of an epidemiologist who traced scarlet fever and of a mineralogist who discovered barium carbonate, he was a breeder of dogs, he played the flute like Jenner, and like Jenner he talked to milkmaids.

Riding through the gentle Shropshire hills in 1775, Withering met an old woman who held the secret of reducing dropsical legs. Limbs bursting from trousers, or lumbering under petticoats, and impossible to shoe, became manageable after her tea of twenty mixed herbs – if you could face the consequent violent vomiting and purging. She cured where the local doctors could not. 'It was not very difficult for one conversant in these subjects,' Withering wrote, 'to perceive that the active herb could be no other than foxglove.' It was the same Godly principle as contained in the scurvy-grass. Nicholas Culpeper (1616–54) had already indicated in 1653 that foxglove 'made up with some sugar or honey, is available to cleanse and purge the body, both upwards and downwards.'

Withering promptly tried the tea experimentally on his patients, the poor ones whom he saw free for an hour every day. It made the dropsical ones pee copiously, an effect overlooked by the old lady of Shropshire. Encouraged by learning that the Principal of Brasenose, Oxford, had been cured by foxglove root of hydrops pectoris (pleural effusion), on 8 December 1775 Withering gave foxglove tea to a builder aged fifty with asthma and fluid in the abdomen, who 'made a large quantity of water. His breath gradually drew easier, his belly subsided, and in about ten days he begun to eat with a keen appetite'.

Unlike the old lady, Withering grasped that the dropsy was pumped away down the Birmingham drains by a heart newly stimulated by foxglove. As 'digitalis', the name since 1542 for foxgloves, the sorcery of Wenlock Edge respectably entered the *Edinburgh Pharmacopoeia* in 1783. Withering's *Account of the Fox-glove* was the enormous success of 1785. He had unknowingly discovered the powerful cardiac drug that, in derivation, is used everywhere today.

Like Jenner, Withering attracted waspish opponents. Dr Lettsom of London killed eight patients with digitalis, including Charles James Fox. Many disasters came from ignorance of dropsy being a symptom, not a disease. It could be caused by a failing kidney as well as by a failing heart. This was established in 1827 by cheerful, chubby, hard-working Richard Bright (1789–1858), the explorer of Iceland, who went from Edinburgh University to Guy's in London. Dropsy at Guy's was still taken as a single illness, as it had been among Withering's Shropshire rustics. But Bright saw a connection between three items: dropsy, the albumen which abnormally appeared in a patient's urine and clouded it on heating, and the hard contracted kidneys at his impending post-mortem. 'After a life of warm affection, unsullied purity and great usefulness', Bright died from heart failure and lives for ever in Bright's disease.

Birth and Death

Lord Lister was handsome, mutton-chopped, gentle, stolid, resolute and impervious to criticism or ridicule. Ignaz Philipp Semmelweiss (1818–65) of Hungary was bald, fashionably moustached, excitable, sensitive and deranged. While Lister was still a student in 1846, Semmelweiss was assistant at the First Obstetric Clinic of the Allgemeines Krankenhaus, Vienna, the biggest lying-in hospital in the world. The First Clinic taught medical students. The Second Clinic taught only midwives. In the First Clinic, puerperal fever a week after delivery, causing bleeding, thrombosis, peritonitis, abscesses, septicaemia and stupor, killed three times the mothers than in the Second Clinic. This was as well known in Vienna as the price of *Bratwurst*, pregnant women in hysterics begging for their confinement in the Second.

Semmelweiss puzzled that puerperal fever simulated another violent disease, that which killed unfortunate doctors who cut their fingers at post-mortems. He reasoned that each mother had a gaping wound: the oozing uterus which had delivered its placenta. He puzzled further over the medical students in the First Clinic coming from the anatomical dissecting-room, while the midwives at the Second Clinic came from their dinners. He decided forthrightly: 'Puerperal fever is caused by conveyance to the pregnant woman of putrid particles derived from living organisms, through the agency of the examining fingers.'

He made the students wash their hands in a disinfectant, chloride of lime. The mortality rate in the First Clinic fell from 18 to 1 per cent. (Reverting to Pasteur, this was seventeen years before he identified these 'putrid particles' as microbes, and nineteen years before Koch matched microbe to malady.) Like Jenner, Lister and Lind, Semmelweiss had cured what he did not know he was curing. The Viennese obstetricians were as unadmiring of his pin-point shot in the dark as were the London surgeons of Lister's.

Lister ended up as a founder member of the Order of Merit, with an Institute, a memorial in Westminster Abbey and a statue outside the BBC. Semmelweiss ended up in a Budapest lunatic asylum, where he died in a fortnight. He had a self-inflicted infection of a finger from his final operation, which made the joint gangrenous, roared through his body and killed him with abscesses of the lungs, exactly like the victims of puerperal fever. Seventy years later, three of every thousand mothers and three of every hundred cases were still dying of puerperal fever. Semmelweiss contained it, but it was the sulpha drugs which eradicated it.

Good Home for a Lost Cause

The summer of 1940 awoke the dreaming spires with air-raid sirens. The war was beginning to bite. We had fumbled nine months through the blackout, and that winter sung 'We'll Be Hanging Out the Washing on the Siegfried Line'. Now butter, meat, tea and petrol were rationed, Scotch was getting difficult, and a fortnight after the war had started properly with the Panzers crossing their neighbouring frontiers, the Germans arrived in Boulogne. In the Drake tradition, cricket continued to be played in the Parks.

To the south of the Parks, in an annex of the Oxford medical school's Pathology Department which usually hutched experimental guinea-pigs and rats, a construction of inverted lemonade bottles, bedpans, rubber tubes, glass pipes, a mahogany bookshelf from the Bodleian, a milk churn, bath-tub, bronze letter-box and electric bell – which would have itched the pencil of Heath Robinson – was manufacturing the most necessary drug of the century.

The Professor of Pathology was Howard Walter Florey (1898–1968), an Australian from Adelaide who looked like Glenn Miller. He had arrived at Oxford from being Professor of Pathology in Sheffield in 1935, and like many an academic new broom swept his young assistants into the Science Library to find neglected or abandoned research worth reviving.

It struck Florey that some work reported by the late Professor Alexander Fleming at St Mary's Hospital in London in 1929 might be worth an experiment. Fleming had been studying the staphylococcus germ, which

69

causes boils, carbuncles, abscesses, wound infection, osteomyelitis, mastitis, pneumonia, septicaemia and death. He had been examining colour changes in the shiny golden staphylococcus colonies, which grow on nutritive agar jelly in the shallow, circular, glass laboratory Petri dishes. These colour changes were more striking if the microbes grew in the open air instead of in the customary incubator.

It seemed that Professor Fleming had gone on holiday in Scotland, with his experiment finished and the infective Petri dishes stacked safely in a bucket of strong antiseptic. But the top dish had mistakenly escaped, and during his month's absence a mould dropped on it and started eating the staphylococci. The late Professor had christened the mould *penicillium* (a brush), and ingeniously used it to clear away from his Petri dishes those irritatingly contaminating germs, like staphylococci and other common ones which caused pneumonia, gonorrhea and diphtheria. Then he could grow the pure *Bacillus influenzae*, which was immune to *penicillium*, which he was studying, which causes sinusitis and bronchitis, sometimes meningitis, but never influenza.

It struck Florey that his deceased confrère's *penicillium* might be re-aimed to attack these common but ferocious contaminating germs inside the body. His German-Russian chemist Ernst Chain (1906–1979) grew the mould on brewers' yeast and extracted its juice, and on 12 February 1941 Florey tried it in the Radcliffe Infirmary, on a policeman with staphylococcal septicaemia following a scratch on the mouth pruning his rosebushes. The penicillin produced on the Bodleian bookcase was so meagre, that they had to bicycle his urine up the road to the Pathology Department for the excreted remains to be extracted and reused.

The patient died, but the experiment was a success. Florey restricted his next life-saving attempts to children: they needed smaller precious doses. His staff planned to smear the mould on their clothes and escape, should the Germans appear in the High. He published his first results in the *Lancet* of 28 August 1940. On 2 September Alexander Fleming (1881–1955) turned up in Oxford, to Florey's surprise. He was not late.

Fleming had all the luck. That Petri dish in St Mary's (viewable in the British Museum) was exposed to one of Britain's horrible Augusts, the low temperature ideal for the mould to grow. The mould itself descended not from heaven, but ascended from the lab downstairs, where the air was thick with moulds because Fleming's colleague was studying them. Fleming was ignorant of penicillin's potential because his mind was curtained, even in the most versatile and inventive microbiological laboratory in Europe under pushy Sir Almroth Wright. For Florey, the curtains had been drawn back. That invading 'everyday' germs could be killed in the blood by chemicals was established in Wuppertal, the month before Hitler took over Germany, by Professor Gerhard Domagk (1895–1964) and several hundred dead mice.

I. G. Farbenindustrie in the Rhineland always made lovely dyes. An obscure Viennese chemist called Gelmo in 1908 had synthesised sulphonamide, which Domagk's boss, the chemist Professor Heinrich Hörlein (1882–1954), swiftly turned into a tenacious and brilliant red one. In 1919, two Americans half-heartedly tried this for killing bacteria in test-tubes, prompted by a German who in 1913 had used a red dye as a skin disinfectant.

It was Professor Hörlein who had the inspiration of sulphonamide as an antiseptic working inside the body. It was the fashionable dream. All over Germany, chemists were synthesising hopeful healing compounds, as busily as their ancestors were identifying bacteria in the 1880s, but without their success. The chemists were animated by Paul Ehrlich (1854–1915) of Frankfurt, discoverer in 1909 of the famous 606 arsenical injection ('The Magic Bullet') to kill the spirochaete of syphilis in the blood. And I. G. Farben chemists had in 1930 already turned a bright yellow dye into the drug mepacrine to kill circulating malarial parasites.

Hörlein set his chemists Mietzsch and Klarer to synthesise innumerable different compounds involving sulphonamide, for Domagk systematically to give to mice which he had infected with twenty-five common bacteria. These included the TB bacillus, gonococcus, pneumococcus, meningococcus, and the streptococcus, which is the germ which caused tonsillitis, scarlet fever, puerperal fever, erysipelas, wound infections and fatal blood-poisoning. All the mice died. Domagk was the archetypical man in the white coat.

In the firm's tradition, I. G. Farben patented sulphonamide. That was on Christmas Day 1932. On Christmas Eve, Domagk had found that twelve mice, infected with streptococci from a human dying of septicaemia, were alive and frolicking. A compound named sulphanilamide had worked.

Domagk won the Nobel prize in 1939, but Hitler did not wish Germans to contaminate themselves with foreign awards, and he was arrested by the Gestapo. Hörlein was arrested by the Americans on 16 August 1945. I. G. Farben made also zyklon-B gas, used by the SS to kill their prisoners. He was tried for his life in Nürnberg in 1947, but got off. The British had meanwhile pinched the patent when war began, and developed the effective anti-streptococcus sulphanilamide into sulphapyridine, which was effective against pneumonia. The penicillin which Florey made in bedpans the Americans made in beer vats, so there was enough for Eisenhower and Montgomery's armies at D-Day. The Americans, like I. G. Farben, patented the process, and henceforth took all the money.

Irony, thy name is progress.

Florey and Fleming shared the Nobel Prize of 1945, but could hardly speak to one another. Then Fleming suddenly confused himself with Robert Bruce. The wee, dry, pawky, inarticulate, incomprehensible Scot toured the world as its saviour, the discoverer of penicillin, and went right to the heart of American clubwomen. Florey retired to magnificent academic solemnity.

Who was penicillin's begetter? Were Florey and Fleming its sperm and ovum? Who remembers what Edwardian grandee physician Sir William Osler said: 'In science the credit goes to the man who convinces the world, not the man to whom the idea first occurs'?

And who remembers the Gloucestershire milkmaids and the Shropshire lads who so knowingly stopped their workaday cuts and bruises going septic by binding them with a slice of mouldy bread?

FOUR

The Conquest of Pain

Anaesthesia was the bright idea of two smart New England dentists on the make.

Laughing Gas and Ether Frolics

Theirs is an oft-told tale. On the Wednesday morning of 11 December 1844, in Hartford, Connecticut, twenty-nine-year-old Horace Wells (1815–48), who was handsome, plump and downy side-whiskered – and was the inventor of a non-tasting solder to anchor false teeth, which failed despite a patients' money-back guarantee – sat in his own dental chair for his colleague Dr Riggs – who was the namer of Riggs' disease, in which all your teeth fall out – to extract an aching wisdom tooth. They had just left the Union Hall, where Gardner Quincy

Colton (1814–98) had by special request given a private exhibition of 'Nitrous Oxid, Exhilarating or Laughing Gas!', which the evening before had provided an entertainment well advertised to be 'in every respect a genteel affair.'

Colton was a failed medical student who lived off popular science. The admirable urge for enlightenment, and the lack of much to do at home in the evenings unconnected with the piano, made such lectures popular, particularly if accompanied with electrical flashes, chemical bangs and convincing stinks.

Nitrous oxide was created in 1772 by Joseph Priestley (1733–1804). He was an embarrassingly impious Presbyterian minister in Birmingham, whose *History of the Corruptions of Christianity* was burnt by the common hangman at Dort in 1785. A Yorkshire cloth-dresser's son with no scientific education, Priestley became the 'Father of modern chemistry ... who never would acknowledge his daughter' (because he clung blindly to the theory of matter containing a mysterious 'phlogiston', the material of fire).

When Priestley accepted an invitation to dinner in July 1791, to celebrate the significance of the fall of the Bastille for Birmingham, a mob wrecked his house, destroyed his papers and smashed his apparatus. He moved to London, to become the morning preacher at Gravel Pit, Hackney, where he found his opinions on the Bible unappreciated and emigrated to Pennsylvania. The year before discovering nitrous oxide, Priestley had extracted from the atmosphere its pure oxygen, which mysteriously made candles burn brighter and mice live longer. He invented soda water.

Sir Humphry Davy (1778–1829) rather liked inhaling nitrous oxide for his headaches: 'A pleasurable thrilling ... vivid ideas passed rapidly through the mind, and voluntary power was altogether destroyed, so that the mouthpiece generally dropt from my unclosed lips.' A West-countryman, Davy was the discoverer of K, Na, Ba, Sr, Ca, Mg and Cl, and was a polished lecturer who ran the fashionable Pneumatic Institute near Bristol. He invented the miners' lamp.

Davy conceived nitrous oxide as useful for surgical operations. But despite his once pinioning patients' limbs and suffering their screams as a youthful surgical apprentice in Penzance, he did nothing about it. He wafted nitrous oxide instead upon Robert Southey, Samuel Taylor Coleridge, and Roget of the *Thesaurus*, who bracketed it with champagne and said it made you feel like the sound of a harp.

Quincy Colton's poster in Hartford enticingly quoted Southey (poet): 'The atmosphere of the highest of all possible heavens must be composed of this Gas'. It made people 'Laugh, Sing, Dance, Speak or Fight, &c, &c, according to the leading trait of their character'. It is always fun to watch people making fools of themselves. Eight Strong Men would fill the front seats to protect the audience from the frenzy of the Twelve Young Men who would volunteer to inhale from the india-rubber bag, and who as an added precaution against vulgarity would be gentlemen of the first respectability.

One such gentleman was Sam Cooley, a drug-store clerk, who gratifyingly went beserk among the benches. Observing wide-eyed afterwards his bloody knees and shins, he exclaimed: 'A man might get into a fight and not know he was hurt.' Adding: 'If a man could be restrained, he could undergo a severe surgical operation without feeling any pain at the time.'

Cooley had uttered anaesthesia's *fiat lux*. Horace Wells sat in the audience. Then a man could enjoy painless tooth extraction under laughing gas? he speculated. The next morning he did. 'A new era in tooth-pulling!' he rightly exclaimed afterwards. As to the man who made a better mousetrap, the world with toothache made a beaten path to his door. After a month, he decamped to Boston to make more money.

His former partner William Thomas Green Morton (1819–68) had studied at the Baltimore College of Dental Surgery and transiently at the Massachusetts General Hospital in Boston, which was founded by John Collins Warren (1778–1856) in 1811. Morton could put Wells on to Warren, who helpfully organised a demonstration for a Harvard student to lose an aching tooth. It was a flop. They all laughed. Wells retreated to Hartford, killed a patient, lost interest in nitrous oxide, gave up dentistry.

We move to Morton's water spaniel.

Ether was 'sweet oil of vitriol' to its discoverer in 1540, the German botanist Valerius Cordus (1515–44). His *Dispensatorium* of 1535 was the first pharmacopoeia, and a best-seller (thirty-five editions). Renamed 'aether' in 1730, the pungent vapour, sniffed, had brought up the phlegm of three centuries. Michael Faraday (1791–1867) in 1818 noticed that ether could stupefy like nitrous oxide, as Morton read in Pereira's *Materia Medica* of 1839. People everywhere were then enjoying 'ether frolics', the alternative to Colton's laughing gas parties, both the ancestors of cocktail parties. Anaesthesia, like drunkenness, was born of mankind's ageless desire to escape from himself, and blessedly escaped infanticide by vicious Puritanism.

Blatantly stealing Wells' idea, Morton tried ether on the dog, who 'wilted completely away in his hands and remained insensible to all his efforts to arouse him by moving or pinching him.' Two minutes later, and the faithful Nig was as frisky as ever! Morton continued experimenting with ether on the dog, on himself, and on his apprentices. It was all deadly secret. He wanted to patent the process and make his fortune.

Morton offered five dollars for a guinea-pig from the

wharves of Boston, but there were no takers. On the evening of 30 September 1846, Eben H. Frost was driven to Morton's surgery by violent toothache, sniffed ether from a pocket-handkerchief, and woke to discover his tooth on the floor.

Sixteen days later, Morton gave ether at the Massachusetts General Hospital for John Warren to excise a veinous tumour on twenty-year-old Gilbert Abbott's left lower jaw. Morton was fifteen minutes late. 'As Dr Morton has not arrived, I presume he is otherwise engaged,' said Warren chillily to the expectant benches of imposing doctors. They all laughed again.

Warren sat, scalpel poised. What drama! Morton hurried in, clutching his brand-new inhaler: a glass globe containing an ether-soaked sponge, with leather flap valves to ensure a one-way flow into the patient's lungs. Success! Warren readdressed the audience: 'Gentlemen, this is no humbug.' End of anaesthesia's Genesis.

The mechanism of Morton's triumph was simple. Ether is far more powerful than nitrous oxide, which is as likely to achieve asphyxia before anaesthesia.

Its good news travelled fast. On the Monday afternoon of 21 December 1846, the first European operation under anaesthesia was done at University College Hospital in north London by lightning-fingered Robert Liston (1794–1847). The surgeon was a six-foot-two Scot who could remove a leg in two and a half minutes. With the patient awake, skilful speed was as great a mercy from the operator as from the executioner. Liston would clamp the bloody blade in his teeth like a butcher, to free his hands and save time, and he proudly notched his amputation knives like Red Indians scored victims on the handles of their tomahawks.

Liston amputated a right leg while Peter Squire, who ran a chemist's shop in Oxford Street, gave ether from a sponge-filled inhaler like a port decanter. 'This Yankee dodge, gentlemen, beats mesmerism hollow,' conceded the vain, abrasive, aggressive surgeon, with powerfully significant generosity. In the painting of this historic operation, luckily the artist not the surgeon removes the wrong leg.

HAIL HAPPY HOUR! WE HAVE CONQUERED PAIN! ran the headlines of the *People's London Journal*. Until that Christmas, mesmerism – after Franz Anton Mesmer from Vienna, the fashionable Paris hypnotist who emitted 'animal magnetism' – or opium, or cannabis, or mandrake, or drink, had been administered to surgical patients, all with more compassion than hope. The Assyrians had produced blackouts by pressing the carotid arteries in the neck. Helen of Troy offered amphoras of nepenthe. The Chinese in 2000 BC pounded rhododendron and jasmine into a sleeping-draught. The Navy gave you a rum-soaked gag, the Army had you bite the bullet. Nothing worked. It was as dispiriting as Florence Nightingale's turpentine tummy rubbings for cholera, and as much of our present treatment for cancer. There was no alternative to courage.

Before springtime 1847, Napoleon's old surgeon Joseph François Malgaigne (1806–65), specialist on the kneecap, had recorded five ether anaesthetics in Paris. Johann Friedrich Dieffenbach, an early plastic surgeon, had administered ether in Berlin. In Edinburgh its innovator was James Syme, Robert Liston's cousin. Nikolai Pirogoff gave ether in St Petersburg, by rectum. The Zurich Council of Health restricted it as dangerous.

That renowned operating speed of surgeons like Pirogoff and Liston – who were compared marvellously to violin virtuosi or duellists – had abruptly become an achievement as outdated as the sedan-chair.

Morton meanwhile needed to hire a secretary. He got hardly any sleep or meals for three months. His medical miracle was all over the newspapers, and the doctors of New England wanted their hands on it. Morton coloured his clear ether fluid and called it 'Letheon'. Anything for concealment, until the patent was fixed. Then he would advertise worldwide, mass-produce his inhalers, present them free to influential surgeons and charitable institutions, and 'send several very costly ones to the chief sovereigns of Europe'. (Fabergé later could have made something of the idea.) Morton wrote pamphlets and engaged salesmen to hire anaesthetic rights from coast to coast. He offered Horace Wells a slice of the action (refused).

Charles Thomas Jackson (1805–80) now turned up. He was a Boston chemist and geologist, and Morton was once his lodger. Jackson invented the electric telegraph before Morse in 1836 and gun-cotton before Schönbien in 1846. He was found mad in 1873.

Morton had prudently if evasively sought Jackson's advice on the chemistry of ether before the adventure of Warren's operation. Jackson now claimed to have suggested the drug himself. He was the true father of anaesthesia, and wanted $500, or 10 per cent of the profits. Morton shrewdly agreed to his sharing the patent. Jackson was of the Boston scientific establishment, and Morton knew that he himself was thought in Boston 'not a man of much cultivation or science' – well, he was thought so by Jacob Bigelow (1787–1879) from Harvard, the botanist and physician who in 1832 saved Boston from cholera (100 dead against 3,000 in New York City). And the jealous Boston dentists were ganging up on him. Partnership with Jackson would be a respectable marriage.

Patent No 4848 was issued on 12 November 1846.

Uproar.

The Boston dentists were outraged at ether becoming 'a secret medicine'. So was the Massachusetts General. 'Many will assent with reluctance to the propriety of restricting by letters patent the use of an agent capable of mitigating human suffering,' haughtily complained Bigelow. Morton caved in. Jackson suddenly remembered the European patents. He demanded a cut, or he would send the Académie des Sciences at Paris a letter claiming his exclusive discovery, by that evening's mail boat. (He sent it, anyway.) Nobody took any notice of the US Patent Office, not even the US Army and Navy in the Mexican war, when Morton offered to etherise casualties at the cut rate of two cents apiece. The net US profits from anaesthesia were to be accounted by lawyers to Morton and Jackson every six months. At the end of the first six they were nil.

Before the finish of his triumphant year, Morton had taken the perennially hopeless, fog-shrouded path of Jarndyce and Jarndyce. He dissipated the rest of his life not in bestowing the benefits of anaesthesia, but in claiming them for himself. He thrice petitioned Congress, which established a Select Committee, which established nothing.

In 1852, Crawford Williamson Long (1815–78) announced calmly that he had been performing superficial surgical operations under ether anaesthesia regularly since March 1842, almost five years before Morton. Long was a popular country practitioner in Jefferson, Georgia. Another country GP had already trailed the scent of anaesthesia: Henry Hill Hickman (1800–30) of Shifnal, Shropshire, had published experiments on puppies with 'suspended animation' by carbon dioxide in 1824. His persistent propounding of gaseous insensibility for surgery in England and in Paris, then the fashionable centre for science, was sadly rebuffed by all from Charles X of France down.

Crawford Long pinned his suspicious disinclination for publicity on native caution, on the scarcity of major operations in a rural practice, and on the risk of confusion with quack mesmerism. But it was added by his daughter: 'It was rumored throughout the country that he had a strange medicine by which he could put people to sleep and carve them to pieces without their knowledge. In case of a fatality he would be lynched.'

Morton took up farming.

On 19 April 1854 the Senate passed a Bill to recompense Morton, on 21 April the House of Representatives rejected it. He was admitted to President Pierce, who concocted a plot for him to sue a government surgeon, instead of the unsueable Government. Morton would win and the Government would pick up the tab. Morton lost, and the Government did not. Morton fell bankrupt, his farm was seized, his family went hungry and ragged, his memories became bitter, his resentment hot, his reputation mocked, his health bad, his life empty. As a diversion, in July 1868 he journeyed from Boston to New York to sue the *Atlantic Monthly*, but dropped dead in Central Park. Wells had meanwhile become a shower-bath salesman, grew addicted to chloroform, was arrested for throwing acid over a couple of Broadway tarts (as John Smith), and on 23 January 1848 bled to death in the Tombs Prison after severing his left femoral artery with his razor. The Paris Medical Society then elected him an honorary member.

His bust is viewable in the place des Etats Unis, near the Arc de Triomphe, alongside a sad plaque still awaiting the statue of World War One General Pershing. It is inscribed: 'Au dentiste Americain Horace Wells inovateur de l'anaesthesie chirgurical.'

French logic is unassailable.

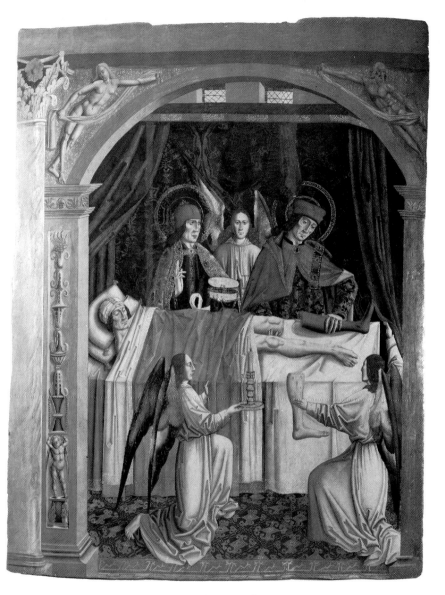

1. *The first transplant:*
saintly surgery by Cosmas and Damian.

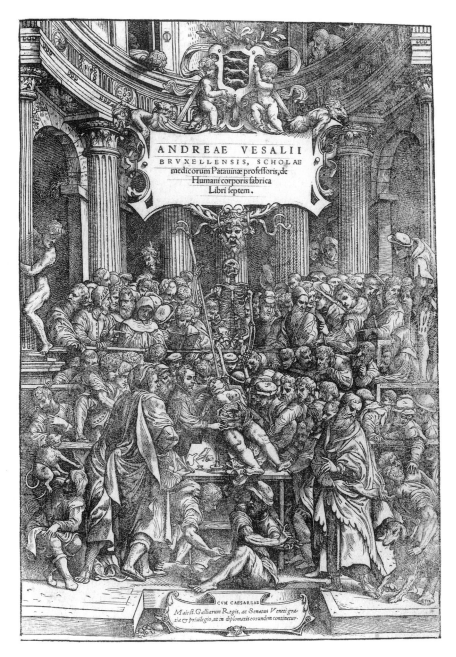

2. Vesalius teaching anatomy.

De mixtura vtriusque sexus seminis, eius que substantia & forma.

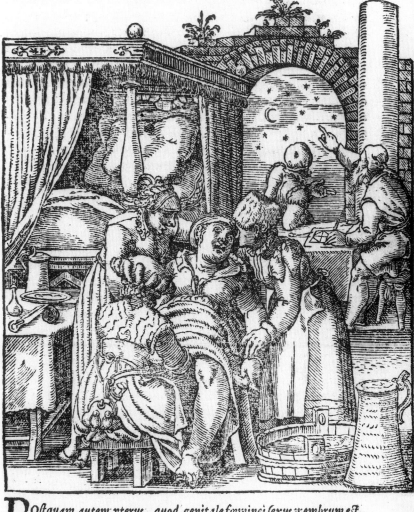

P Ostquam autem vterus, quod genitale foeminei sexus membrum est,
viri genituram conceperit, suum quoque semen illi admiscet, ita vt ex
ambobus

3. *Domiciliary delivery, mid-sixteenth century.*

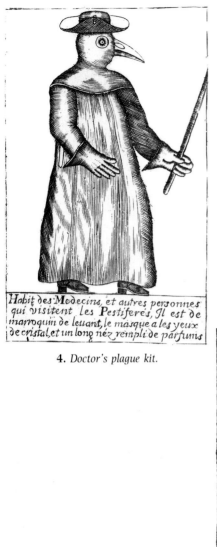

Habit des Medecins, et autres personnes
qui visitent les Pestiferés, Il est de
marroquin de levant, le masque a les yeux
de cristal, et un long néz rempli de parfums

4. *Doctor's plague kit.*

5. *Weight watching, 1614.*

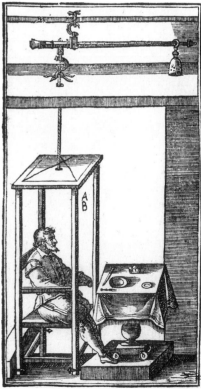

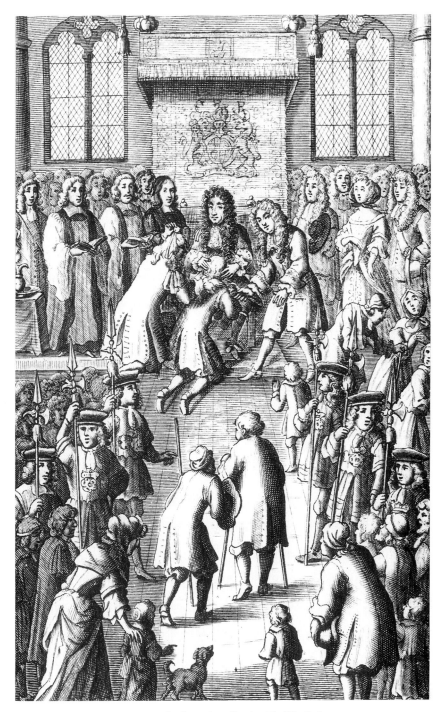

6. *A touch of royalty: Charles II's TB clinic.*

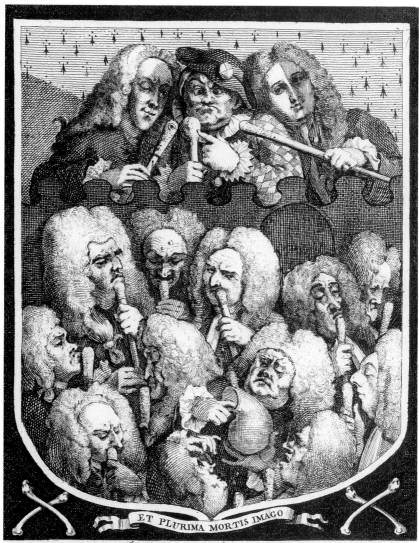

ET PLURIMA MORTIS IMAGO

The Company of Undertakers

Beareth Sable, an Urinal proper, between 12 Quack-Heads of the Second & 12 Cane Heads Or, Consul-
-tant. On a Chief Nebulæ, Ermine, One Compleat Doctor issuant, checkie Sustaining in his
Right Hand a Baton of the Second. On his Dexter & Sinister sides two Demi-Doctors, issuant
of the Second, & two Cane Heads issuant of the third; The first having One Eye conchant, towards the Dexter Side of the Escocheon; the Second Faced per pale proper & Gules, Guardent. —
With this Motto ———— Et Plurima Mortis Imago.

* A Chief betoken ith a Senatour or Honourable Personage, borrowed from the Greeks, & is a Word signifying a Head; as the Head is the Chief Place in a Man, or the Chief in the Escocheon should
be a Reward of such only, whose High Merits have procured them Chief Place, Esteem, or Love amongst Men. Guillim.
** The bearing of Clouds in Armes (saith Upton) doth impart some Excellency.

Price Six pence

Publish'd by W. Hogarth. March the 3d. 1736

7. Hogarth's doctors, sniffing their gold-headed canes
and tasting their patients' urine.

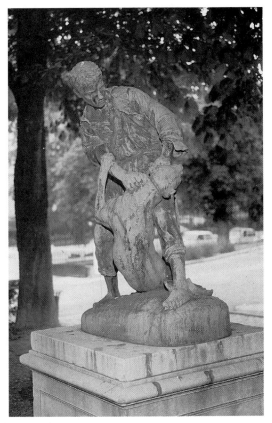

8. *Juptile and the mad dog in the Institut Pasteur, Paris.*

9. *Europe's first anaesthetic. Liston is performing the operation (on the wrong leg).*

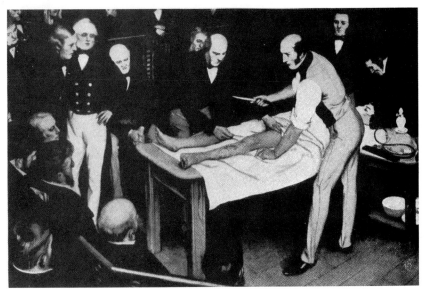

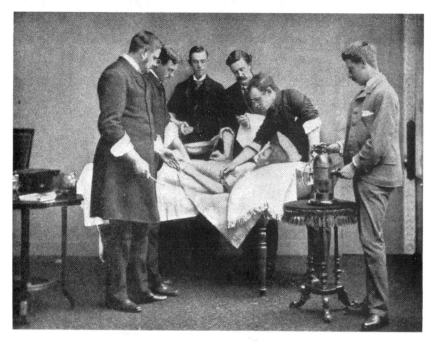

10. *Lord Lister's carbolic spray.*

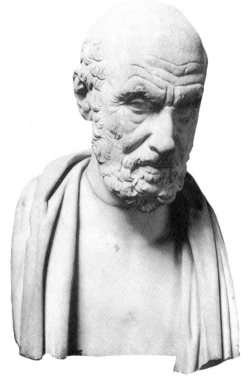

11. *The father of medicine, Hippocrates.*

Chloroform and Religion

Sir James Young Simpson, Bt (1811–70), seventh son of a baker, Professor of Midwifery, *accoucheur* to the carriage trade, Queen Victoria's Physician in Scotland, hallowed by a private chapel built into his squat granite house overlooking the Firth of Forth, attracted a practice worth £80,000 a year to the local hotels. He was an Edinburgh Festival right round the calender.

After dinner on Thursday 4 November 1847, Sir James partook with his two young assistants from the Edinburgh Royal Infirmary chloroform instead of port. Inhaling the bouquet, the pair of junior doctors burst into laughing, shouting, and attempting to hurl the chairs and dining-table through the windows, then slid snoring to the floor. 'Far stronger than ether,' observed the bulky professor, following them down.

Ether's blissful honeymoon had ended. Its stink, its irritation of the lungs, its vomiting patients, the necessity for awkward glassware and to use gallons of the stuff, sent doctors seeking to perform the magic of anaesthesia with other wands. Chloroform was quick: a blow rather than a bludgeoning into unconsciousness. It smelt nice and lasted longer, it was powerful, cheap and simpler to give. Just sprinkle it on a nightcap or a worsted glove. Soak a bath-sponge in it, and you could cut off anything. Half a teaspoonful of chloroform, dripped on a handkerchief folded over the nose, exorcised the labour pains that had bedevilled mothers since Eve, and outraged the (male) clergy of Scotland.

'In sorrow thou shalt bring forth children', directed Genesis. To 'rob God of the deep earnest cries' of a mother in labour, they preached, ensured her never loving the child for which she had never suffered. Ah, yes! countered the equally pious Simpson (who kept two family Bibles in his dining-room). But surely the next verse directed man to eat in sorrow all the days of his life, yet everyone seemed to enjoy their haggis and bashed neeps?

The elders quibbled about the translation of 'sorrow'. He corrected them: 'It signifies not sensations of pain but the severe muscular efforts of which human parturition consists, the uterus being more powerful, and the mechanical obstacles to birth being more numerous, than enjoyed, for example, by the domestic cow.' The cow did not do. These menacingly righteous and dangerously well-meaning people (who are ever with us) continued dissenting until 7 April 1853, when John Snow (1813–58) administered chloroform *à la reine* to Queen Victoria for the painless delivery of Prince Leopold and afforded Genesis respectability.

As Jackson in Boston snatched at the credit for ether from Morton, so a bald, bushy-bearded Scottish surgeon turned chemist, David Waldie (1813–89) reached for the garlands laid upon Sir James Simpson. Chloroform is an unsophisticated compound: $CHCl_3$, as simple as ether's $(C_2H_5)_2O$, and the even simpler C_2H_5OH of man's universal casked or bottled joy, alcohol. Chloroform was concocted in 1831, independently in Paris, Germany and New York State. It was tried as an anaesthetic on animals by the French physiologist Pierre-Jean-Marie Flourens (1794–1867, he discovered the centre which regulates breathing in the brain) nine months before Simpson experimented on himself. It had already made lots of people drunk in New York.

Simpson heard about chloroform from Waldie, chatting at the Edinburgh Medico-Chirurgical Society that October 1847. Waldie worked for the Apothecaries' Company in Liverpool, and had looked up its formula in the United States Dispensatory to oblige a local doctor, who was trying it to bring up the phlegm of Liverpool instead of ether. Waldie promised Simpson a sample, but got home to find his lab burnt down. When Simpson proclaimed to the world chloroform (bought from Duncan and Flockhart off Princes Street) within a week of his anaesthetic dinner-party, Waldie found himself a rankling footnote.

The resentment outlasted the life of the detractor. 'He had a greater share in the introduction of chloroform than Dr Jackson had in the introduction of ether,' declared John Snow – damnably faint praise. Waldie died still sore but rich in Calcutta, after which his native Linlithgow put things right with a plaque: 'To him belongs the distinction of having been the first to recommend and make practicable the use of chloroform in the alleviation of human suffering.'

They were resentful, too, seventy miles to the south in Dumfries. Robert Liston's removal under ether of the right leg of a thirty-six-year-old Harley Street butler in University College Hospital had grabbed the London publicity. But on the Saturday before that, the first operation under anaesthesia in Europe had been unnoticeably performed in the Dumfries and Galloway Royal Infirmary, administration by William Fraser (1819–63), surgeon aboard the Cunarder *Acadia*, which had docked in Liverpool at 9.15 am, three days earlier, bringing the glad news of Morton's performance from Boston via Halifax. Perhaps they all deserved Simpson's amicable advice: 'Never nurse a grudge. It's as uncomfortable as a cold hot water bottle.'

Chloroform soon ousted ether everywhere. Though unwitting sadists persisted into Florence Nightingale's heyday: 'The smart of the knife is a powerful stimulant, and it is better to hear a man bawl lustily than to see him sink silently into his grave,' ordered Sir John Hall (1795–1866), principal medical officer in the Crimea.

W. E. Henley appreciated in the 1870s:

Behold me waiting – waiting for the knife.
A little while, and at a leap I storm
The thick, sweet mystery of chloroform,
The drunken dark, little death-in-life.

And its easefulness at both ends of the operation was indicated by George Bernard Shaw in 1906:

Chloroform has done a lot of mischief. It's enabled every fool to be a surgeon.

Evaporation of Chloroform

There was a snag about chloroform. It killed people swiftly, unaccountably and indiscriminately. The first victim was Hannah Greener, fifteen and perfectly healthy, at Newcastle on 28 January 1848, having a toe-nail removed. Too much chloroform would of course kill you, like too much anything else. But it was soon discovered that the heart could stop suddenly early in the administration – 'chloroform syncope'. Nobody knew why. This caused a dreadful row in Hyderabad on 25 January 1889.

The Duke and Duchess of Connaught were distributing prizes at the medical school of this far-flung academic outpost of the Empire upon which the sun never set. Its Principal (Bengal Army Medical Service) boasted it was a better medical school than a lot of European ones, and they had anyway discovered that 'there is no such thing as chloroform syncope'. They did this by killing with a straightforward overdose 128 full-grown pariah dogs. He advised London medical schools to stick to ether, which they knew how to manage.

The *Lancet* was incensed. Letters and leaders clashed masterfully in the weekly issues which sailed out aboard the P&O mailships. The Nizam of Hyderabad sportingly put up £1,000 for the *Lancet* to send an expert to test their theory. The *Lancet* dispatched an eminent pharmacologist, who wired back NONE WHATEVER HEART DIRECT after killing 490 dogs, horses, monkeys, goats, cats and rabbits. The *Lancet* snootily suggested their own man had gone native. As repeatedly in medicine, the doctors continued to argue and the patients continued to die.

Chloroform is uninflammable, while ether is explosive, which recommended its use in battles and air-raids. In World War Two, it was superseded by an uninflammable dry-cleaning fluid, trichlorethylene (cleaners were delightedly getting drunk by sniffing the tanks). After the war, like Rowntree's Motoring Chocolate and Stop-Me-And-Buy-One ices, chloroform never made a comeback.

The Rag and Bottle

Anaesthesia has produced more ingenious pieces of apparatus even than horticulture. John Snow was the world's first professional anaesthetist. A Yorkshireman, the eldest of a farmer's nine children, he lived in Soho and worked at St George's Hospital at Hyde Park Corner, giving ten anaesthetics a week. In 1847 he invented a portable ether inhaler the size of a thick book, which contained a water-bath to vaporise the anaesthetic, which was poured into a chamber containing a spiral baffle-plate, from which the patient inhaled the heavier-than-air vapour by a long flexible tube. A valved triangular mask covers the mouth and nose – in Snow's monograph, of a pretty girl with delightful ringlets. Snow applied a scientific mind to a novel subject that had emerged from chance and speculation, and could easily have been lost in superstition and quackery. He wrote *On Chloroform and Other Anaesthetics*, dropping dead on finishing the last paragraph.

Joseph Thomas Clover (1825–82), bushy-bearded and frock-coated, followed Snow as London's sought-after anaesthetist. He practised at the Westminster Hospital and included in his patients Sir Robert Peel, the former Napoleon III, the future Queen Alexandra and Miss Florence Nightingale, possibly in order of intimidation. He invented a chloroform inhaler, by which a dose from a syringe was vaporised and pumped by a bellows into a shoulder-bag the size of a pillowcase, all of which terrified nervous patients. This provided $4\frac{1}{2}$ per cent chloroform in air, the first anaesthetic to be measured. He invented also 'Clover's crutch', for keeping the anaesthetised patient's legs in the air while the surgeon got at the perineum.

The anaesthetic apparatus which littered the second half of the nineteenth century varied from a simple wire-and-flannel mask which you carried about in your top hat, to an ornamental reservoir like a teashop urn for the nitrous oxide that was returning to dental favour. Some had bulbs like scent-sprays for pumping air through a bottle of chloroform, some had handles driving cogwheels, many had rubber bags like footballs, but Frenchman Louis Ombrédanne (1871–1956) used a pig's bladder.

His compatriot Paul Bert (1830–86) invented in 1879 the anaesthetic car, sturdily air-tight, lit by ten portholes, with room for twelve people, including the patient. The operating team was subjected to high-pressure air, and the patient to high-pressure nitrous oxide from a bag billowing under the operating table. The air was refrigerated in summer and delivered through hot water in winter, and if it ran short someone inside blew a whistle to the man outside at the pump. The car ran on neat wheels and was moved round the Paris hospitals, until in 1883 the passengers succeeded in directing it to the scrap-heap. The doctors were luckier than the three balloonists whom Paul Bert dispatched aloft to study life-saving oxygen inhalation, only one of whom landed alive.

After World War One, anaesthesia was generally accomplished by running compressed nitrous oxide and oxygen from cylinders across ether, or sometimes chloroform, poured into jam-jars. This was the simple invention of 'Cocky' Boyle (1875–1941), who with 'Gloomy' Hewer (1896–1986) embellished anaesthesia from St Bartholomew's Hospital in the City of London. Sir Ivan Magill (1888–1986) had anaesthetised during the war for Sir Harold Gilles, who invented plastic surgery at Sidcup. To save the battered face becoming a battleground for surgeon and anaesthetist, Magill deftly slipped a tube past nose, palate, tongue and vocal cords into the windpipe. Thus there was no impediment between the bottom of his life-sustaining oxygen cylinder to the spongy alveoli composing the patient's lungs. This was a welcome convenience for anaesthetists, who spent much time and struggle preventing their patients from choking themselves.

Despite the gadgets, and their necessary augmented expertise, the anaesthetist remained the genially despised 'rag-and-bottle-man', bottle of chloroform in one tail pocket of his morning coat, square of lint to drip it upon in the other, recipient of ten per cent of the surgeon's fee, the Figaro, the Admirable Crichton, the Jeeves of the operating theatre.

The Academic Accolade

In 1937, Europe's first anaesthetic professor was thrust among the others at Oxford, to their outrage. The money came from Lord Nuffield, who had already outraged Oxford in its entirety with his locally mass-produced Morris Minor motor-car ('Oxford is the Latin quarter of Cowley,' it was chic to sigh). Nuffield was blackballed at the local golf club, so he bought it, and installed his golfing partner in the anaesthetic Chair. This was Sir Robert Reynolds Macintosh (1897–1989), inventor of the improved laryngoscope, who had already proved his ability by administering a faultless dental gas to his benefactor. Sir Robert ran an efficient Harley Street practice involving three gas-machines and two Bentleys per anaesthetist, enviously called after the prewar institution 'The Mayfair Gas, Fight and Choke Company'. Then the National Health Service made anaesthetists consultants like anyone else, they founded the Faculty of Anaesthesia, and at last arrived at the hospital driving the same sort of car as the surgeon.

America already had a professor, Ralph Milton Waters (1883–1979) at Madison, Wisconsin. He introduced cyclopropane gas, with the disadvantages of its being horribly explosive and horribly expensive. Also 'Pentothal', which changed the terrifying induction of anaesthesia from controlled suffocation to just one little prick in the arm, my dear. (If the anaesthetist could unerringly make the vein: 'Did you have gas for your operation?' asked the woman on the bus. 'No, they don't give you gas any more,' her friend replied. 'A bloke comes and sticks a needle in the back of your hand four or five times, and then you go off to sleep.')

'Locals' were used since 1884, either injected into the flesh, or picking off nerves, or knocking out the spinal cord itself, or simply smeared on the surface of eye, tongue or nose. The magic power of cocaine was famously exploited by the Viennese eye surgeon Carl Koller (1857–1944), who pinched the idea from his friend Sigmund Freud. Had Freud not gone on holiday with his fiancée at the time, he might have become an acclaimed pioneer anaesthetist, and saved the world much agonising introspection.

Local anaesthetics were widely used because they produced numbness and paralysis without the bodily upset of a narcotic drug, and without the need of a skilled anaesthetist. But a 'local' is obstinately local, and riskier oblivion is generally the patient's preference. The solution was provided by Sir Walter Raleigh (1552–1618). Voyaging to the Orinoco in 1595, Sir Walter reported the paralysing arrow poison of the South American Indians, a syrup from a creeper later named 'curare'. The world's operating tables are now filled day and night with people suffering the equivalent of a hit by a poison dart from a blowpipe. The patient's paralysis offers the surgeon flaccid rummaging, while an innocuous trace of some modern anaesthetic like halothane offers superficial sleep. The anaesthetist is particularly stingy during Caesareans, through fear of harming the baby, sometimes with the alarming result of a conscious and utterly paralysed patient throughout. The courts are so famously bountiful in compensation of such physical and mental agony, that any mother complaining of the experience may suddenly recall to a whole maternity ward that they, too, suffered undeservedly.

This epic combination of sleep and paralysis which transformed anaesthesia was ventured by Harold Randall Griffith (1896–1985) at Montreal in 1942. But French novelist Joris-Karl Huysmans thought of it first. Writing in 1884, about Edgar Allan Poe's remarks on the depressing influence of fear upon the will, Huysmans adds:

> Which it affects in the same way as anaesthetics
> which paralyse the senses and curare which cripples
> the motory nerves.

Well, well.

Nobody knows why anaesthetics work. But nobody knows why we fall asleep.

FIVE

The Gold-headed Cane

The seventeenth-century physician was useless but decorative. Satin gilt-buttoned coat, buckskin breeches, silk stockings and buckled shoes, lace ruffles, full-bottomed wig, swinging a long cane with a hollow gold head filled with an aromatic Marseilles vinegar. This was *le vinaigre de quatre voleurs*, the clearly efficient concoction of four arrested, but uninfected, plunderers of dead bodies in a Marseilles plague. It was repeatedly sniffed to afford the doctor security from infection, and time to think. The cane became his symbol, the magic wand of Aesculapius.

Pomp and Sad Circumstance

The Gold-headed Cane of 1827 is the gossipy autobiography of an arms-emblazoned cane carried successively by five fashionable physicians after 1689. First was John Radcliffe (1650–1714), who bestowed upon Oxford the Radcliffe Camera, the Radcliffe Library and the Radcliffe Infirmary. He was physician to William III, who was grumpy, drank a lot, and gobbled up the rare green peas without ever offering any to the Queen. Royal treatment was difficult, bleeding the King requiring assent of the Privy Council. Arrogant Radcliffe had a row with Sir Godfrey Kneller over a shared garden door: 'Sir Godfrey might do even what he pleased with the door, so that he did not paint it.' To which the artist replied through his footman: 'Tell Dr Radcliffe that I can take anything from him but physic.' Well, they chortled over it in the Mitre Tavern in Fleet Street, where Radcliffe was lavish on his vast £5,000 a year (later, Sir Godfrey got the picture).

The guinea had come in with the Restoration, conveniently rounding up the doctor's fee from a noble, 6s 8d. Though unminted after 1813, the guinea persisted as the genteel unit of medical currency until decimalisation in 1971. Travelling expenses by carriage were an extra. To be seen by a London doctor in Pitlochry cost 1,500 guineas. Radcliffe fell in love when he was sixty, and got lampooned. When Queen Anne was dead he was gouty, and Parliament blamed him for not attending her, but he made reasonable excuse by dying himself three months later.

'I have never read Hippocrates in my life,' Radcliffe sullenly told a young doctor, who had inquired politely if he read Hippocrates in the Greek. 'You, sir, have no occasion,' the youngster replied promptly. 'You are Hippocrates himself.' Thus Richard Mead (1673–1754) fixed for himself inheritance of Radcliffe's practice and gold-headed cane. Mead initiated healing by post, writing prescriptions at half-a-guinea a time at Tom's Coffee House in Covent Garden, without troubling to see the patients. In the evenings he moved to Batson's. He made

£7,000 a year. 'Dr Mead,' said Dr Johnson, 'lived more in the broad sunshine of life than almost any man.'

The cane which smoothed the palms of these gold-fingered doctors is now in the Royal College of Physicians. This was founded by Thomas Linacre (1461–1524), a Fellow of All Souls, Oxford, who achieved letters patent establishing proper physicians from Henry VIII in 1518, a twenty-two-year jump ahead of the surgeons. The College was empowered to oust from medical practice the thriving charlatans, monks, artificers and women who brought 'grievous hurt, damage and destruction to many of the King's liege people; most especially to them that cannot discern the uncunning from the cunning.' Really empowered: in 1630 and 1637, it cut two unlicensed practitioners' ears off. The Bishop of London was appeased by being allowed to continue licensing doctors as freely as ordaining priests. The Royal College of Physicians, with the gold-headed cane viewable, is now near the Zoo.

Other worthy decorators of two centuries' medicine:

- Dr Johnson's own doctor, William Heberden (1710–1801), who described angina pectoris and Heberden's nodes (arthritis on the fingertips).
- Eccentric, strict Quaker Thomas Hodgkin (1789–1866) was thought at Guy's not at all the sort of chap they wanted to join them on the consultant staff. He settled for being Curator of the hospital Museum, where he discovered, in pathological specimens, a simultaneous enlargement of the spleen in the abdomen and of the lymph glands scattered all round the body. Nobody took any notice of this correlation for thirty-three years, until Guy's physician Sir Samuel Wilks (1824–1911) resurrected it, and very decently named it Hodgkin's Disease.
- The deafness and giddiness of an ear disease was described by Prosper Menière (1799–1862), of the Paris Institution for Deaf-Mutes, a month before he died of influenza.

- Sir William Withey Gull, Bt (1816–90), physician to Queen Victoria, sensibly suspected the efficiency of all drugs and wrote *Rheumatism Treated by Mint Water*. He got the Prince of Wales through typhoid (there was no treatment) and dropped aphorisms:

Not a typhoid fever, but a typhoid man. (The doctor treats a patient, not a disease.)
Savages explain, science investigates.
Of a difficult neurotic: Mrs X is herself multiplied by four.

A century later, Sir William became the butt of lunatic accusations by the straining legatees of our folk hero, Jack the Ripper. That ghoulish autumn of 1888 Gull was seventy-one, he had suffered an ischaemic attack of the brain the year before, and he endured arthritis of his Napoleonic frame. Which suggests that he found more comfortable ways of spending his evenings than dodging round the gaslit alleys of Whitechapel vigorously slicing up tarts. He left £344,000, a medical record.

- Yorkshireman Sir William Richard Gowers (1845–1915), was the neurologist who first brandished the peep-show opthalmoscope to view the informative retina of the eye, he also defined Gower's tract in the spinal cord.
- Sir Hans Sloane (1660–1753), the physician who had an exotic garden in Chelsea and founded the British Museum, named Sloane Square, Sloane Avenue and Hans Crescent, all on the route to Harrods, also Sloane Rangers.

Diagnosis Is All

Victorian physicians were brilliant at identifying all the diseases that they had no idea how to cure.

- *Percussion*. Musical Leopold Auenbrugger (1722–1809), son of a Graz innkeeper, applied the finger-tapping which discovered the level of wine in his father's casks to discover the level of fluid in a diseased chest. This appeared outrageously undignified to his fellow Viennese physicians. Jan Nicholas Corvisart (1755–1821), Napoleon's physician, thought this a splendid idea, which in 1808 he spread round Paris – like Sir Samuel Wilks, *honorablement* giving credit to its author.
- *Auscultation*. To hear the heart beating and the lungs rustling, every doctor since Hippocrates had simply applied ear to chest. This method was described by René Théophile Hyacinthe Laënnec (1781–1826) as 'not only ineffective but inconvenient, indelicate, and, in hospitals, even disgusting'. Doctors were known to have laid their head upon a soft bosom, and in a matrimonial way dropped off to sleep. So Paris in 1816 produced another lasting diagnostic aid, when Laënnec was confronted by a girl with such enormous tits he impulsively rolled up a handy quire of paper, listened from a seemly distance, and invented the stethoscope. This was at first a wooden cane, then an ear-trumpet, then the familiar double-eared equivalent of the magic gold-headed cane.
- *The Pulse*. Counting the pulse accurately was tricky before watches had second-hands. Ex-medical student Galileo (1564–1643) timed his pendulum from his pulse, then cleverly inverted the idea by timing his pulse from his pendulum. A fellow professor at Padua, Sanctorius Sanctorius (1561–1636), in 1625 invented the pulsilogium, a pulse-watch, which after two centuries was improved in Lichfield by Sir John Floyer (1649–1734), so that it ran for a minute. Sanctorius spent much of his life sitting in a weighing-machine observing how much he put on after meals, anticipating the twentieth century's science of metabolism and obsession with slimming.
- *The Temperature*. Galileo had invented a thermometer, Sanctorius improved it for human use,

but it was a foot long and needed sucking for twenty minutes. Scholarly Sir Thomas Clifford Allbutt (1836–1925), the original of George Eliot's Dr Lydgate in *Middlemarch*, reduced it to something which nurses could poke into their top pocket. Carl Reinhold August Wunderlich (1815–77) of Württemberg invented the temperature chart, and in 1868 became enlightened that the raised bodily heat which it recorded was not itself, as everyone thought, an illness: 'He found fever a disease and left it a symptom.'

Benjamin Rush (1745–1813), the Hippocrates of Pennsylvania, a Quaker, anti-war, slavery, hanging and alcohol (views good for his practice), was a signatory of the Declaration of Independence and declaimed: 'Medicine is my wife and science my mistress.' ('I do not think that the breach of the seventh commandment can be shown to have been of advantage to the legitimate owner of his affections,' commented Dr Oliver Wendell Holmes of Boston.) Rush became enlightened that inflammation was the *effect* of a disease, rather than the *cause*. Between them, Wunderlich and Rush enjoyed two glittering visions of infection, before practical microbiology at the end of the nineteenth century rendered them as unremarkable as photographs.

– *X-rays*. Wilhelm Konrad Röntgen (1845–1922), Professor of Physics at Würzburg in Bavaria, working late on the Friday night of 8 November 1895, noticed that some distant crystals in his dark laboratory became illuminated as electricity passed through the vacuum tube he was using inside a black cardboard cover. He shifted the crystals further away. They still lit up. He put a book between. A piece of wood. Then metal plates. They still shone. He stuck his hand in the way. *Mein Gott!* The bones showed through. He got the Nobel Prize in 1901. Röntgen was a simple, sad, dreamy, modest man, who hated the publicity, gave Nobel's 50,000 kroner to his University, refused to call them Röntgen rays or to cash in commercially, told everyone that the Kaiser would lose the war and died alone and broke.

Pierre Curie (1859–1906) and his Polish wife ex-children's governess Marie Sklodowska Curie (1867–1934) in 1897 discovered radium. Pierre was run over in the Paris traffic, and Marie died of anaemia from exposure to radium.

A Piece of Antique Furniture

Amid the gently-creaking leather upholstery, the clink of ice on crystal, the soft rustle of *The Times* in the gentlemen's clubs of Pall Mall, are strange pieces of ancient furniture unidentifiable even by the oldest members. The velveted and tasselled gout stool, tucked under the cushion of the commodious club armchair, allowed a swathed toe, so excruciatingly tender that the alighting of a buzzing fly was anticipated with alarm, to be raised into the blissful horizontal.

Many diseases have clubs, with addresses and telephone numbers, from Alcoholics Anonymous and Arthritis Care to Venereal Diseases. Some lingering illnesses became informal clubs, a camaraderie among the members compensating for their gloomy untreatability. In the earlier twentieth century, the TB sanatoriums up Swiss mountains offered the comradeship of a regimental mess in a war with an uncomfortable casualty-rate. Gout was the clubbable affliction of gentlemen. The hobbling, bandaged, crutched, fat, red-faced, ill-tempered, porty sufferer inflamed the imagination of Gillray, Rowlandson and everyday cartoonists like their own big-toe joints.

It was ill-matched mockery. Sir Thomas Browne discovered in the mid-seventeenth century: 'What famous men, what emperors and learned persons have been severe examples of that disease, and that it is not a disease of fools, but of men of parts and senses.'

Six admirable sufferers from this historical complaint:

- Byron. ('Gout, which rusts aristocratic hinges.')
- W. S. Gilbert. ('A taste for drink, combined with gout, Had doubled him up for ever.')
- Jaroslav Hasek, *The Good Soldier Svejk*. ('The Colonel . . . was suddenly transformed by a fit of gout from a gentle and peaceful lamb into a roaring tiger . . . he roared in the frightful voice of a man who is being slowly roasted on a spit: "Get out everybody! Give me a revolver!" ')
- Sydney Smith, wit. ('I observe that gout loves ancestors and genealogy. It needs five or six generations of gentlemen or noblemen to give it its full vigour.')
- James Thomson, poet. ('The sleepless Gout here counts the crowing cocks, A wolf now gnaws him, now a serpent stings.')
- Anthony Trollope. ('Old gentlemen generally are cross. Gout, and that kind of thing, you know.')

Gout is clearly an affliction of the literary.

There was gout in the skeletons of AD 3 in the Cotswolds. The Romans swallowed a gouty propensity with the lead from their drinking-vessels. 'Poor men seldome have it,' *The Haven of Health* was noticing in 1584. This was because the poor lived on barley bread and cheese, while the gouty classes ate the protein which fuelled their disease. The port was the fire-lighter.

Thomas Sydenham (1624–89) wrote *A Treatise on the Gout* in 1683, describing: 'The victim goes to bed and sleeps in good health. About two o'clock in the morning he is awakened by a severe pain in the great toe . . . so exquisite is the feeling of the part affected, that it cannot bear the weight of the bedclothes nor the jar of a person walking in the room. The night is passed in torture, sleeplessness . . .' The doctor wrote with such clinical insight because he suffered horribly from gout himself.

Sydenham, from Wynford Eagle in Dorset, was a graphic raconteur of all diseases. Sydenham's chorea, 'St Vitus' dance' occurring in streptococcal-infected children, was one of his originals. He shrewdly differentiated measles from scarlet fever: 'The measles generally attack children . . . disquietude, thirst, want of appetite, a white (but not a dry) tongue . . . on the fourth day there appear on the face and forehead small red spots, very like the bites of fleas.'

White tongue? Perhaps it is fanciful that Sydenham observed also those white and helpfully diagnostic early white spots in the mouth, two centuries before Henry Koplik (1858–1927) of Mount Sinai Hospital in New York.

Sydenham is flattered as 'the English Hippocrates', because he rubbished the theories, mysticism and magic that festooned contemporary medicine. He reincarnated the Hippocratic idea of treating the patient at the bedside, from what he himself saw, and from what he himself knew. He preferred *Don Quixote* to medical textbooks. And he had the supreme clinical gift of recognising when he could do his best for his patient, and for his reputation, by doing nothing whatever.

His ardent pupil was pirate-physician Thomas Dover, who got smallpox and had Sydenham's fever treatment of cold room, fresh air, no bedclothes and twelve bottles of small beer every twenty-four hours. For consumption, Sydenham prescribed horse-riding. He distributed opium to everyone, tastily mixed with saffron, cinnamon and cloves. Sydenham was modest, unimpressionable, aloof, compassionately 'answerable to God' for his patients. He had been one of Cromwell's captains of horse, and he enjoyed the admirable Cromwellian quality of sniffing the whiff of bullshit in the winds of history.

After Sydenham, British foreign policy established gout officially in 1703, with the Methuen Treaty. This was to woo the Portuguese away from France, by a £7 a tun duty on port against £55 on a tun of claret. English gentlemen could then afford to drink four bottles of port a night, having nothing better to do in the evenings, after finishing the latest volume of *Pamela*, except chatting over the dinner-table until disappearing under it.

With the laudable social equality of our age, gout is now available to 6 in 1,000 of the British people.

The Methuen Treaty was annulled in 1835.

The Fevered Brow

Three of medicine's pivots were not doctors. Charles Darwin was a sea-going naturalist, Louis Pasteur was an industrial chemist, and Florence Nightingale was a nurse.

Florence Nightingale (1820–1910) is legendary for the wrong reasons. Even the Lady's lamp is wrong, illuminating either our old £10 note or the pedestrian crossing to the front door of the learned gentlemen's Athenæum Club in Pall Mall. Along the four miles of corridors that composed the wards at Scutari she swung a linen Turkish Army lamp, crinkled like a Chinese lantern, a candle throwing an orange glow at the base. Miss Nightingale's other fist grasped the three essentials of politics: knowing what she wanted, knowing whom to get it out of, and knowing how long to wait for it. She could have run the country as ably as Lord Palmerston, had she not returned from the Crimea and gone to bed for fifty years. She had numerous other peculiarities, like angrily slamming the open lids on lavatory seats.

As Churchill's destiny was set on course as First Lord of the Admiralty in 1911, Miss Nightingale was launched by The Institution for the Care of Sick Gentlewomen in Distressed Circumstances, No 1 Harley Street, the year before the Crimean War. She was its Superintendent, with the touch of Snow White among the Seven Dwarfs. She promptly fired the resident doctor, ordered the groceries wholesale from Fortnum's and the vegetables by the sack from Covent Garden, she made her own jam, installed food-lifts, hot water and patients' bells, killed the rats, mice and bedbugs, and stopped the gas exploding. In six months, Miss Nightingale halved the sick gentlewomen's running costs. She had a way of getting her way: 'If a repair is not done I will encamp with my twelve patients in the middle of Cavendish Square and let the police and the Committee come and rout me out as a vagrant.'

She could not possibly have been anything but an Englishwoman. The Nightingales of Embley House in Hampshire were stylish travellers (Florence was born in Florence, she could as easily have been called Rimini), and London socialites (half a floor of the Carlton Hotel for the Season, two daughters presented at Court). Miss Nightingale knew Sidney Herbert, the Secretary *at* War (not *of*, he kept the books). Brisk politicking got from Lord Aberdeen's Cabinet her unanimous promotion from Harley Street to Superintendent of the female Nursing Establishment of the English General Hospitals in Turkey, and within a week she was off from Dover with forty nurses.

Miss Nightingale immediately reorganised the hospital, which had been created by the Army by whitewashing the inside walls of the Selinie Barracks at Scutari. This is a huge building, its corners crowned with four towers, visitable across the Bosporus from Istanbul (Turkish sweet *paklava* is delightful, and *raki* makes a change from gin-and-tonic). Miss Nightingale scintillated the brighter from the rest of the war not being organised at all. She next organised the clothing and feeding of the local British Army by spending *The Times'* £30,000 fund in the Constantinople bazaars, having already organised the British Ambassador, who had earmarked the money for building a local Protestant church.

When pain and anguish wrung the brow, Miss Nightingale had far more important things to do than be a ministering angel. She continually organised the burials of her patients – also their letters home – but left the dirty work in the wards to the dirty nurses. These were women she thought: 'Who were too old, too weak, too drunken, too dirty, too stolid, or too bad to do anything else.' Her own nurses had sailed from Dover to the unthinkable for 12s a week, plus a pint of porter for dinner and a glass of Marsala at supper. Three years after the Crimean War, Miss Nightingale's orders to them appeared as *Notes on Nursing*, a slim volume with the end-papers of its 1895 reprint advertising the equally practical *Pig-Sticking or Hog-Hunting* by Capt Baden-Powell, *Cricket, Jerks in from Short Leg*, by Quid, and Bailey's railway conveniences, male and female.

Some of her jottings:

- Don't make your sick-room into a ventilating shaft for the whole house.
- Absurd statistical comparisons are made in common conversation by the most sensible people for the benefit of the sick.
- Averages of mortality tell us only that so many per cent will die. Observation must tell us *which* in the hundred they will be who will die.
- Help the sick to vary their thoughts.
- Patient's repulsion to nurses who rustle. On which Miss Nightingale expands:
- I wish too that people who wear crinoline could see

the indecency of their own dress as other people see it.
A respectable elderly woman stooping forward,
invested in crinoline, exposes quite as much of her
own person to the patient lying in the room as any
opera dancer does on the stage. But no one will ever
tell her this unpleasant truth.

The light of genius is perceptible in gleams. She wrote
also *Notes on Nursing for the Labouring Classes.*

In bed in South Street, Mayfair, Miss Nightingale
organised the Army Medical Department, the Nightingale Training School for Nurses at St Thomas's Hospital,
and the sanitation of India. Visitors called from the
Cabinet Room, our embassies, episcopal palaces, and
from Buckingham Palace with the Order of Merit, catching her just before she died. One visitor was from Oxford:

> First come I; my name is Jowett.
> There's no knowledge but I know it.
> I am Master of this college:
> What I don't know isn't knowledge.

Who wanted to carry her off to Balliol and marry her.

Some years ago, I wrote a novel indicating that Miss
Nightingale, from her own declarations at the age of 41
('I believe I am "like a man" . . . My experience of women
is almost as large as Europe. And it is so intimate too. I
have lived and slept in the same bed with English
Countesses and Prussian country girls . . . No woman
has excited "passion" among woman more than I have')
was a lesbian. Such finger-pointing has since become a
popular game in the literary playground. Lesbianism is
as irrelevant to someone of Miss Nightingale's qualities
as a sensibility to draughts. It brought her one advantage.
It stopped her marrying Jowett.

Muliebrity was a traditional necessity in caring for the sick. For curing them, it was more doubtful. Sir William Jenner (1815–98) – the physician who worked the donkey-engine to spray Queen Victoria's armpit with Lister's carbolic, and squirted the Queen in the face – was sobbing away during Miss Nightingale's resplendent middle age that he had only one dear daughter, but he would rather follow her bier to the grave than see her become a medical student. Lister himself raised an objection to christening the new Lister Professor of Surgery at Glasgow: 'Considering the relations the new Chair will have to do with the teaching of women.' The rest of the necessarily sensible medical profession made less fuss about death being preferable to learning to prevent it.

Elizabeth Blackwell (1821–1910), the daughter of a religious sugar-refiner with a household of nine children and four maiden aunts at Bristol, emigrated to New York when she was eleven. At twenty-six, after rejection by Philadelphia and other medical schools across the United States, Miss Blackwell got into Geneva Medical College, NY. She graduated top of the class, so setting a pattern in academic application that women in medicine have found difficult to shake off. Her initial difficulty was finding lodgings, landladies shuddering at providing a bed for an unchaperoned girl. In 1857, Elizabeth Blackwell founded the New York Infirmary for Indigent Women, run by women. She commanded the nurses in the Civil War. Unmarried, she adopted an orphan.

Elizabeth Garrett Anderson (1836–1917) was the first lady of British medicine, and Sophia Jex-Blake (1840–1913) among the first Scottish (though in Edinburgh, women were genteelly segregated for teaching). By World War One, lady doctors became commissioned officers in the British Army, with pips on their cuffs like the gentlemen. Now British women medical students outnumber the men. And if women complain of discrimination in specialties like surgery, that is through the inescapable biology of a male surgeon taking only a few seconds to create a baby, but a female one manifestly longer. The Church of England is meanwhile suffering a ludicrous neurosis about women priests, which beneath the theological, liturgical and social arguments expresses the well-founded fear of Sir William Jenner's abettors: that the girls might show them up.

The Start of Medicine

Physicians ventured into the twentieth century lightly armed. They bore mercury for syphilis and ringworm, digitalis to strengthen the heart, iodine for goitre, colchicum for gout, chloral for the excitable, a pomegranate alkaloid for tape-worms. Since 1867 they had amyl nitrite for angina, and it was Thomas Sydenham who first prescribed iron for anaemia. The thick textbooks of 1900 are as sweepingly accurate on diagnosis as today's, but the chapters are all tragedies because they lack a happy ending of effective treatment.

Claude Bernard (1813–78), from whose father's vineyards flowed Beaujolais, when a young druggist's assistant at Lyons wrote a musical comedy *La Rose du Rhône*, which did so well at the box-office that he turned seriously to drama by writing the five-act *Arthur de Bretagne*, which he presented for the opinion to the Parisian critic Saint-Marc Girardin, who advised him to take up medicine.

Bernard was a laboratory doctor, a thoughtful experimenter: 'Put off your imagination, as you take off your overcoat, when you enter the laboratory; but put it on again, as you do your overcoat, when you leave.' In 1857 he discovered that the liver produced sugar, independently of the sugar which the liver's possessor ate. So the body's organs were not a diverse bundle, each functioning to destroy and excrete ingested chemicals. They could create their own chemicals, through which the organs could act one upon another. Bernard called it *le milieu intérieur* – the weather existed inside us as well as out. This introspection breezed endocrinology into medicine.

Claude Bernard also deposed the stomach as the monarch of digestion, and installed the pancreas as its powerful prince. He investigated pancreatic function by implanting a cannula in a stolen dog, which escaped home to its owner, who was a police inspector. The anti-vivisectionists of 1850 henceforth disagreed that the exceptional intelligence and original conceptions of Claude Bernard should be so allowed to benefit present and future humanity. Luckily, the reconciled police inspector stood up for him. Bernard's wife did not understand him, either.

Ivan Petrovich Pavlov (1849–1936) was an equally skilful experimenter, whose discovery of a dog's salivation at the sight or smell of its din-dins, or even at the ringing of its dinner-bell, named the oft-adapted Pavlovian 'conditioned reflex.' Though the fame should belong to Diderot, who described in *Rameau's Nephew* a century earlier:

> He had a mask made like the face of the Keeper of the Seals, he borrowed the latter's ample robe from a footman. He put the mask over his own face. He slipped on the robe. He called the dog, caressed it and gave it a biscuit. Then, suddenly changing his attire, he was no longer the Keeper of the Seals but Bouret, and he called his dog and whipped it. In less than two or three days of this routine, carried on from morning to night, the dog learned to run away from Bouret the

Farmer-General and run up to Bouret the Keeper of the Seals.

Musical Glands

Dubliner Robert James Graves (1796–1853), a man of action who was jailed in Austria as a spy and quelled a mutiny in the Mediterranean, had observed in 1835:

> Violent and long continued palpitations in females, in each of which the same peculiarity presented itself, viz: enlargement of the thyroid gland . . . the eyes assumed a singular appearance, for the eyeballs were apparently enlarged, so that when she slept or tried to shut her eyes, the lids were incapable of closing.

Evermore, we had Graves' disease from an over-active thyroid.

The pituitary gland at the base of the brain later became 'the leader of the endocrine orchestra', a seven-piece ensemble. It was Harvey Williams Cushing (1869–1939), Professor of Surgery at Johns Hopkins and Harvard, who struck up the band. He began sorting out the pituitary in 1912, and described its moon-faced Cushing's syndrome in 1932.

Thomas Addison (1793–1860), a grocer's son, a rude man who came from Newcastle to Guy's in London, in 1849 gave his name to a fatal anaemia without a cause, 'pernicious' anaemia. On 15 March 1855, he described to the South London Medical Society a second Addison's disease, a disorder of the suprarenal endocrine glands which brought pigmentation of the skin and a risk to life. This was the unheard overture of the endocrine orchestra. Addison had the misfortune, shared with Guy's man Thomas Hodgkin, of being so far ahead of his time that nobody took any notice. He developed melancholia and shortly died in Brighton.

By 1935, physicians were equipped with injections of liver as ammunition against pernicious anaemia. In 1922, Sir Frederick Banting (1891–1941) and Charles Herbert Best (1899–1978) of Toronto armed them with insulin to treat diabetes. They could still fire off Sir Gowland Hopkins' vitamins, and snipe with Sir Almroth Wright's inoculations.

Medicine was slowly shaking off its Victorian values of diet, regular bowel movements, beef-tea and rest and quiet, a regimen so restful that for some sickly women it meant immobility for three months, flat in bed without callers, newspapers and letters, the only relief the barrel-organ at the end of the street. Luckier patients were dispatched on sunny holidays or voyages, a convenient route for a perplexed doctor to get rid of them.

Until the second half of the twentieth century, the physicians' pharmacy remained largely a magazine of blank cartridges. Now thrived the medical armourers. We have today effective antibiotics, antihypertensives, anti-arrhythmics, anti-emetics, antidepressants and anti-convulsants, also steroids against arthritis, bronchodilators, diuretics, healers of stomach and duodenal ulcers, endocrine regulators and replacements, drugs against Parkinsonism and cytotoxic drugs against cancers. The leukaemias of childhood have lost their terror, and some savagely fatal diseases – like seminoma of the testis – released of their malignancy. We live longer and feel better. The effect of this victorious advance is less universal jubilation than widespread complaint, inspired by our politicians, that winning this war is bankrupting the National Health Service and making the drug companies a fat profit.

Since 1799, the Greene King brewery of Bury St Edmunds has nourished Cambridge undergraduates with Abbot Ale. It flows delightfully at the Eagle Pub in Botoph Lane, convenient for the Cavendish Laboratory and the Medical School facing it across Downing Street, where the more perceptive inhabitants of both went for lunch. The medical students thought the Cavendish's physicists and chemists a weird mob, which was one of the world's many speculations confirmed by the discovery of the double helix of the molecule of DNA.

The structure was described in 1953 by American James Dewey Watson (b 1928) and Englishman Francis Harry Compton Crick (b 1916). The idea was not new. It dates from 1519. François I of France, the year before meeting Henry VIII on the Field of the Cloth of Gold, started building the Château de Chambord. From the middle of the guardroom in the donjon rises a magnificent spiral staircase of two superimposed helices, which never meet. The hub has decorative openings, to see from one helix into the other. It may be pleasantly observed on a day's tour of the Châteaux of the Loire (Muscadet is excellent value, and the local *rillettes de porc* are highly agreeable before the essential Loire shad *au beurre blanc*).

The double staircase in Cambridge had two twisting handrails of sugar-phosphate on the outside, the steps composed of the bases adenine, thymine, guanine and cytosine, bonded together in pairs by hydrogen, which represents the spindle up the middle. The flight is called DNA, deoxyribonucleic acid. RNA is the slightly different ribonucleic acid, its messenger. RNA is the pattern for the proteins which form the body's cells, of varying design but all furnished with DNA staircases.

The finding of DNA's architectural skeleton made a

fascinating, light-fingered, erudite thriller, written by James Watson in the *genre* of Dorothy Sayers at the time. The characters are:

- (1) Himself. The intruder from Chicago in the cosy, cold-shouldering cloisters of Cambridge. Breathtakingly clever, ambitious, impetuous, intuitive, charmingly *gauche*, sociable, with a flair for foreign travel.
- (2) Francis Crick from Mill Hill in London, a fast and loud talker with a thunderclap laugh, deep in the theories of protein structure, nagged by Watson to pursue ploddingly the ideas which flocked from his brain. Just remarried, living next to Cambridge's only Chinese restaurant.
- (3) Maurice Hugh Frederick Wilkins (b 1916), biophysicist at King's College in the Strand in London. Bachelor and English gentleman.
- (4) Rosalind Franklin (1920–58). The Dark Lady of the Chromosomes. Newnham, then research on coal. Specialised early in x-ray crystallography, which was usually applied to metals and to minerals. Used this technique to investigate DNA, independently, in Maurice Wilkins' King's laboratory, which accepted women scientists with the baffled dutifulness of wartime farmers receiving Land Girls. Daughter of a wealthy Jewish banking family, she lived in smart South Ken and travelled abroad third-class with little money, to pit her wits against the world. Unmarried, unloved, and seemingly unliked.
- (5) Linus Carl Pauling (b 1901), Professor of Chemistry at the California Institute of Technology, Nobel Prize runner, McCarthy victim, the unseen threat.

The plot was the race to solve the DNA mystery, which everyone was frightened that the powerful and rich American Pauling might win. It involved fascinating jealousies, duplicities, conspiracies, vanities and theatricalities. Watson hated Rosalind Franklin's dresses and blue-stocking dowdiness, complained about her scorning make-up and hairdos, and thought that she was bad-tempered, intolerant and grim. He assiduously called her 'Rosy', to her infuriation. He comforted himself in the Cavendish 'that the best home for a feminist was in another person's lab'.

On Jim Watson's paying a call at King's in the Strand:

> Suddenly Rosy came from behind the lab bench that separated us and began moving towards me. Fearing that in her hot anger she might strike me, I . . . hastily retreated to the open door.

Assault – who knows, murder? – was averted by the gentlemanly intervention of Maurice Wilkins. Such unseemliness would never have occurred among doctors, though a Presidential Address to the Royal Society of Medicine in 1963 mentioned fisticuffs between Sir Peter Freyer and Hurry Fenwick over controversial methods of removing the prostate.

The Cavendish Professor of Physics was Sir William Lawrence Bragg (1890–1971), who had won the Nobel Prize for x-ray crystallography in 1915. Like any deeply settled laboratory head, he must have preferred a quiet life to the squabbles and enthusiasms of his clamant juniors, whose work he knew from weary experience could equally well turn out world-shattering or worthless. Sir Lawrence felt, however uncomfortably, obliged to contribute a foreword to Watson's sniffy book *The Double Helix*, to which he accords 'a Pepys-like frankness.' Clearly, he was a master of donnish understatement.

Watson won the race. Or was he pipped at the post? Rosy's x-ray investigation of DNA crystals began unravelling its molecular structure between January 1951 and June 1952. On 6 February 1953 Wilkins (rather ungentlemanly) passed one of Rosy's x-rays to Watson, who exclaimed: 'Look, there's the helix, and that damned woman just won't see it.' So perhaps it was Rosy who first hit the reproductive idea of the century. But in the excitement nobody bothered to ask. She never got over it. She died of cancer in the spring of 1958, aged thirty-seven. Thirty-four years later, English Heritage put a blue plaque on her flat.

The Double Helix was briefly proclaimed by Watson and Crick in a 900-word paper in *Nature* in April 1953. Though Crick had already announced 'We have found the secret of life!' most appropriately over Abbot Ale at lunchtime in the Eagle.

Genes

Genetics is a subject as opaque and as boring as theological philosophy, but similarly contains the secret of eternal life.

- Inheritance lies in the chromosomes, contained in wavy dark hairs, obvious down the microscope, within the blob of nucleus in every cell.
- These hairs hold forty-four paired chromosomes, and two more: an X plus an X chromosome in females, an X plus a Y chromosome in males.
- All cells in any body have the same number of identical chromosomes: apart from the sex cells, which have half as many. When these males and female sex chromosomes meet up, after the male and female have, if the X takes a fancy to the Y they have a boy, if to an X a girl.
- Chromosomes consist of genes.
- Genes are composed of varying lengths of double helix DNA. They are groups of many nucleotides, which are chemicals consisting of nitrogen, pentose sugar and

phosphate. The order of these nucleotides differentiates one gene from another.
— Every body's genes are different from everybody else's genes, except identical twins.

The number of cells in the body is three followed by twelve noughts, an awful lot. The DNA in each cell is about two metres long. If you untwined it all, it would reach to the moon and back 8,000 times. It is rather thin. Geneticists are fond of offering this information to show what a difficult subject they have inherited.

Nevertheless, geneticists are starting to make a map, called a genome, showing which genes reflect various diseases. Each abnormal gene, responsible for its particular disease, is always on the same place on its chromosome. So they can pinpoint the gene causing, for example, sickle cell anaemia, on every chromosome they look at. Enthusiasts can move about with a syringe taking family blood samples at weddings and funerals.

Throw-back to Darwinism

As Lister discovered antisepsis knowing nothing about streptococci, and Lind cured scurvy while knowing nothing of vitamin C, so Darwin founded genetics knowing nothing about DNA.

Charles Robert Darwin (1809–82), spent five years from Christmas 1831 sailing the South Seas in the 242 ton, 90-foot long, three-masted *HMS Beagle*, which is the size of a yacht belonging to a minor millionaire. As he had seventy-three shipmates, it must have been highly uncomfortable. He sailed from Devon to Rio, rounded Cape Horn, and called at New Zealand and Australia before rounding the Cape of Good Hope, then homeward bound recrossed the South Atlantic to Brazil before reaching Falmouth on 2 October 1836. On 16 September 1835 Darwin landed in the Galapagos Islands, on the Equator in the Pacific, and there saw eternity in the finches.

Galápago is Spanish for tortoise, of which the Islands had alarming ones the size of crustacean prize pigs. There are a dozen Galapagos islands, which Darwin explored for a month. He discovered excitedly that the reptiles, birds, fish, insects and plants of the Galapagos were slightly different from those anywhere else. They even differed from island to island. The finches had strong short beaks to crack the nuts on one island. Delicate beaks to catch the insects on another island without nuts. Thicker beaks to feed on the fruit offered by yet another island. Longer beaks to nose out the grubs on a fourth. The finches existed through their beaks, which were evolved over generations of finches to eat what was going. Darwin brooded there was something in all this.

He retired ashore on an inheritance of £5,000 a year to a vast house at Downe in Kent beyond Orpington (visitable, good local pub). There he passed twenty-three years thinking over the finches of the Galapagos before publishing *On the Origin of Species by Means of Natural Selection* in 1859. He was jogged by the unexpected threat materialising the previous June of losing his glory to Alfred Russel Wallace (1822–1913), a naturalist who had hit on the same idea. It was like Rosy and Watson.

A suspicion that the world's animals and plants were not identical replicas of originals out of the heavenly workshop had been lurking in human minds since Babylon (where they were interested in the varying manes of horses). The minds included those of Bacon, Buffon, Goethe, Lamarck, Herbert Spencer and Sir Charles Lyell. Lyell was a geologist, who gave Darwin the idea of interpreting the continuing present from the evolving past, as in rocks. Genetic ideas occurred also to Augustinian monk Gregor Johann Mendel (1822–84) of Moravia, who crossed the varieties of garden peas which he sowed in 1853 in Brno, and which blushed unseen in the scientific air until the end of the century. And to Darwin's own grandfather, Dr Erasmus. Darwin had in the meanwhile married a first cousin and fathered ten children, seven surviving, and developed hypochondria.

Darwin's confirmation that Sir Thomas Browne had the right idea 225 years earlier, by his suggesting in *Religio Medici* that Genesis was not as reliable as the Victorians' railway timetables, was taken as an affront of science to the Church. This culminated on 30 June 1860, amid uproar with sobbing and fainting ladies, in the University Museum beside the Parks at Oxford.

The Church had a case. Everyone knew the world was created in 4004 BC, at 9 o'clock on the Sunday morning of 23 October, it had been worked out a couple of centuries earlier by the Archbishop of Armagh and the Vice-Chancellor of Cambridge University. So whose word did you take? Darwin's? Or the Word of God?

'Soapy Sam' Wilberforce, Bishop of Oxford, was out 'to smash Darwin' at the thirtieth annual meeting of the British Association for the Advancement of Science, which was conveniently held on the episcopal doorstep. He sarcastically dismissed a hostile doubter: 'Is it through Mr Huxley's grandmother or grandfather that he claims to be descended from the apes?' This pince-nezed scientific wasp, Dr Thomas Henry Huxley (1825–95), replied: 'I should most certainly rather be descended from an ape than from a man who prostitutes his education and his eloquence to the worship of prejudice and falsehood.' Such ya-boo was thought as shocking as flicking ink-balls in the upper sixth of the late Dr Arnold's Rugby. One of Darwin's detractors that Oxford tea-time was Vice-Admiral Robert Fitz Roy, ex-captain of *Beagle*, who had read a paper on 'British Storms' and now brandished his Bible at his former shipmate in violent anger, and five years later cut his own throat.

Darwin's thoughts linger with us. Sufferers from sickle-cell anaemia have developed out of the survivors from malaria. And there are white people and black people in the world, because people with black skins take longer than people with white skins to create – from the sunlight – vitamin D inside them. Lack of vitamin D causes disabling rickets and osteomalacia. When man moved from the Equatorial sun to the chilly north seeking food, only the paleskins could survive and multiply, becoming paler and paler. (This may be rubbish. Asian ladies in Britain become brittle-boned from consuming chapattis, which contain phytate, which prevents the absorption of vitamin D from their guts. Though this may be rubbish, too. Such are alarming amusements of medicine.)

The Alarming Future of Medicine

Modern science has brought the world the possibility of speedy evolution through practical genetics, as it brought the possibility of its speedy total destruction through atomic weapons.

We now grab diseases by their molecules. The gene can be identified which causes – for example – inherited sickle-cell anaemia. Or haemophilia or cystic fibrosis. Or Huntington's chorea, which gives perfect health in youth, then condemns its inheritor to ten years of stumbling dementia and death. All these unborn victims can be spared by abortion, or possibly prevented by genetic choice of marriage partners. 'Having observed the mating habits of my fellow men for some years, I am not optimistic about the future of this approach,' decided the Oxford Professor of Medicine, Sir David John Weatherall (b 1933). Adding, equally sagely, to the patients-must-decide lobby: 'Parents (and patients) come to doctors for help, and the counsellor must sometimes be prepared to offer positive advice, in order to assist as well as to share in their decision making. Indeed, the sensitive clinician will often notice the relief that parents show when some of the burden of decisions as onerous as this is taken from them.'

The fault, dear Brutus, is not in ourselves but in our genes that we are mortal. It is melancholy medicine that our effort to prevent some diseases is futile and muddled. Cigarettes and alcohol kill, so can gluttony and sloth, but many overweight people reach old age without performing any exercise beyond lifting the elbow and flicking the lighter. We are now spotting the genes which carry diabetes, cancer of the colon, hypertension, hardening of the arteries. Soon we shall seize and eject those provoking other 'everyday' diseases. Later, we shall be able to implant desirable ones. If a couple desire red-haired sons as musical as Mozart and as intelligent as Einstein who can play cricket like Jack Hobbs, no trouble. Man gropes for the ultimate ability to control his environment and himself. Utopia looms.

This will become a matter of such importance to humanity that television programmes will be made of it. Commissions will be convened of the great and the good, who want to become greater and better. Important people will express their deeply held beliefs and prejudices, which are often interchangeable. Politicians to whom eternity is the next election will sow flowery opinions to gather votes. Tolerance will be happily exploded by those familiar worthy organisations who confuse the importance of human life with their own. Like abortion and embryo research, moral compromise will evolve with laws to save man's face in the belief that they are saving his soul. Our intelligence creates problems which our intelligence cannot handle. Come back Socrates, we're sorry about the hemlock.

SIX

The Demon Barbers

Modern surgery was invented by gunpowder.

Battle Honours

Through the inexorable advance of civilisation, sword-thrusts and arrows were superseded around 1450 by powder and shot. Its advantages were instantly recognised. It was a more labour-efficient way of mutilating and killing humans, which invited ingenuity in its application, and which necessitated implements that were soon cheap to produce in profusion. It swiftly accomplished the end of the Hundred Years' War and of Feudalism. It later confirmed both the superiority of Americans over Red Indians, and the nineteenth-century European ownership of Africa, by its particular effectiveness in the hands of the few against the many without it.

The ravages of gunpowder occupied Renaissance surgeons equally with those of syphilis. Shots and sores were the commonest obvious blights on mankind. A sword or halberd opens up the body with a clean sweep, but gunshot complicates military assault with burning flesh and bits of lead and leggings left inside. Queen Elizabeth I luckily retained astern of Hawkins and Drake her army surgeon Thomas Gale (1507–86), whose *An Excellent Treatise of Wounds made with Gonneshot* contradicted all Europe's other surgeons in 1563, by noticing that the dirty bullet was *not* as hot as the purifying cautery. Her Majesty was equally well served at sea against the Armada by William Clowes (1549–1604), who in 1591 said the same thing in *A Profitable and Necessarie Book of Observations for All Those that Are Burned With the Flame of Gunpowder Etc and also for Curing of Wounds Made with Musket and Caliver Shot and Other Weapons of Warre Commonly Used at this Day both by Sea and Land*.

The succeeding French kings François I (who died in 1547, aged fifty-three), Henri II (who died in 1559, after a wound during a friendly joust with a Scotsman), François II (who married Mary, Queen of Scots aged fourteen, and died from an ear abscess aged seventeen in 1560), Charles IX (who died of TB, aged twenty-four, in 1574) and Henry III (assassinated aged thirty-eight in 1589) were even more fortunate at this innovative time to enjoy as their army surgeon Ambroise Paré (1510–90), the Father of Modern Surgery.

The current treatment of gunshot wounds was pouring on boiling oil, but one night during François I's assault on Turin in 1537 Paré's oil ran out, so he applied instead an emulsion of eggs, rosewater and turpentine. After an anxious and sleepless night himself, Paré was relieved to find next morning these patients alive, *et tant mieux!* barely touched with pain and fever. His boiling oil patients were swollen, agonised and dying. Paré henceforth eschewed boiling oil, added to his mixture puppy-fat, worms and oil of lilies, and went round saying humbly 'Je le pansay, Dieu le guarit' – I applied the dressing, God applied the cure.

Paré was another irrepressible medical aphorist. Two are worth lodgement in a medical student's mind:

- Always hold out hope to the patient, even if the symptoms point to a fatal issue.
- He who becomes a surgeon for the sake of money will accomplish nothing.

Paré was another practical doctor like Hippocrates, who preferred learning from his patients, not his books. In the ten days between Henri II's jousting wound and death, Paré puzzled out the best treatment by dissecting four fresh human heads, kindly donated by local criminals. A suspected Huguenot, he survived the St Bartholomew's Day massacre in 1572 through protection in the chamber of their royal slaughterer. 'It is not reasonable that one who is worth a whole world of men should be thus murdered,' conceded Charles IX. Paré mercifully abolished castration as the routine cure of male hernias.

A Surgical Benefactor

Warfare remained an admirably consistent stimulus to the development of surgery. The bigger and better the wounds, from the steady improvement of their causative technique, the abler and more knowledgeable became the surgeons. The specialty thus owes much to Napoleon. The Emperor himself was wounded in his campaigns but once, at the Battle of the Pyramids in 1798, when he was kicked on the foot by his horse. His surgeon was Dominique Jean Larrey (1766–1842), 'the most virtuous man I have ever known', to whom he left 100,000 francs, and made a baron for his butchering officers' horses to feed the wounded.

Larrey invented the 'flying ambulance', a light box on two well-sprung wheels drawn by a pair of horses, to collect wounded from the battle instead of leaving them to die until it was all over. As surgeon-in-chief to *la grande armée* Larrey led a busy life (1,900 wounded at Aboukir, 200 amputations a day at Borodino). He was wounded himself at Waterloo, became surgeon to Louis-Philippe, and was waiting at Les Invalides in his Wagram uniform when Napoleon came home from St Helena.

On the other side at Waterloo was Sir Charles Bell (1774–1842), a Scotsman moved to Soho Square, expert artist and fly-fisherman, the anatomical separator of the motor from the sensory nerves, which matched Harvey's discovery of circulating blood. He is popularly remembered by Bell's one-sided palsy of the face. He was the son of the Manse, lived well, and died impoverished.

Sir Charles operated impartially upon friend and enemy, with two hours' sleep a night:

> It is impossible to convey to you the picture of human misery continually before my eye . . . While I amputated one man's thigh, there lay at one time thirteen, all beseeching to be taken next . . . It was a strange thing to feel my clothes stiff with blood, and my arms powerless with the exertion of using the knife!

Eight days after the Battle he visited the battlefield:

> The view of the field, the gallant sorties, the charges, the individual instances of enterprise and valour

recalled to me the sense the world has of victory and Waterloo. But this is transient. A gloomy, uncomfortable view of human nature is the inevitable consequence of looking upon the whole as I did – as I was forced to do.

Indeed.

Surgery has repaid the inspiration of warfare by making it less lethal. The splint to immobilise broken limbs, designed by a Welsh bone-setter's son, chain-smoking, cloth-capped Hugh Owen Thomas (1843–91), a GP in the Liverpool slums, was introduced for compound fractures of the femur in 1916, and by 1918 had reduced their mortality from 80 to 20 per cent. The Kaiser's uncle, surgeon Friedrich von Esmarch (1823–1908), insisted on kit-bag field-dressings in the Franco-Prussian war of 1870–71. He invented a vast rubber bandage to squeeze all the blood from a preoperative leg, making life easier for the surgeon. Nikolai Ivanovitch Pirogoff (1810–81), the Russian ether innovator, was a military surgeon who mirrored Florence Nightingale in the Crimea by irritating the authorities, insisting on medical comforts and introducing female nurses.

In World War One, the United States forces suffered 234,300 wounded, of whom 14,500 died of their wounds. So 219,800 wounded survived, 6.25 per cent. In World War Two, the United States Army alone had over twice as many wounded, 572,027, and 25,493 of them died of wounds, 4.5 per cent.

A more comfortable way of killing your fellow-man is by car. The British government department in charge of designing and controlling roads was proud that the latest 4,655 annual deaths from road accidents had fallen to the level of forty-three years ago. On British roads in 1930, 4 per cent of those injured died. In 1960, 2 per cent of those injured died. In 1990, 1.6 per cent died. So surgery makes safer drivers, too.

All the King's Surgeons

The history of surgeons is more encouraging and consecutive than that of physicians, because they were a bunch of barbers who went snipping and shaving more adventurously. Ambroise Paré had come from the textile town of Laval, the son of a barber, the brother of a barber, and a barber. In 1500, Paris enjoyed the keenly snobbish distinction between these barber-surgeons and the academic 'surgeons of the long robe'. It was the same socially in the days of Madame Pompadour, between the upstart *noblesse de robe* and the feudal *noblesse d'épée*. The University of Paris Medical Faculty, which had been added to Divinity, Arts and Law in the twelfth century by Louis VII, upped the standing of the barbers in 1503 by embracing them, not the long-robed surgeons, whom it hated. These had to slink off and try to join the physicians. The Paris physicians, *ca va sans dire* despised surgeons of any sort.

The barbers of clubable England had formed guilds in all the cities, like the Grocers and the Drapers and the Haberdashers, and rose socially when Thomas Vicary (1495–1561) persuaded his patient Henry VIII to declare them all surgeons. His Majesty graciously established the United Barber-Surgeon Company in 1540 (Holbein got the picture). This was fundamentally a trades union closed shop, with the perk of two hanged criminals a year for practising anatomy. It sported the enduring red-and-white striped barber's pole, symbolising bandaging and bleeding. The Scots won a similar charter in 1506 from James IV, but only one criminal a year, though they got the Edinburgh whisky monopoly.

After almost 150 years, the London surgeons began to feel that barbers were not at all the sort they cared to mix with, and they petitioned Charles II for a divorce. This was eventually granted by George II in 1745, when they became the new Company of Surgeons, built Surgeons' Hall in the Old Bailey, and started eating their agreeably convivial dinners.

Pott's Unfortunate Fracture

1756 was a busy year for London town planners. Westminster Bridge had been opened as London's second in 1750 (Canaletto got the picture) and Pitt Bridge was programmed to start in 1760 (though it became Blackfriars). South of the Thames, new roads were outlined radiating from Lambeth Marshes: once off the Lambeth Horse Ferry, go straight on past the Archbishop's Palace, then turn right at the Dog and Duck for the Kennington Turnpike and Surrey; or turn left past the Fishmongers' Almshouse for the Old Kent Road, Canterbury, the Channel ports and the European community.

The King's three-hour passage from Whitehall to Greenwich Palace would be sensationally speeded to three-quarters. The tolls: a penny a coach, ha'penny a horse. Percival Pott (1714–88), surgeon to St Bartholomew's Hospital – which faced upon the Smithfield Cattle Market in the City – was riding during the January of that foreseeing year up the Old Kent Road, to cross London Bridge for his home in Bow Lane, when he fell off his horse, sustaining Pott's fracture.

The treatment for open fractures was necessarily ruthless: amputation. Lying in the muck surrounded by gawping Londoners, Pott eyed the two spiky halves of his tibia poking through the skin of his lower leg. With professional impassiveness, he dispatched a messenger across the river to Westminster, for a pair of sedan-chairmen to hasten along with their poles. He meanwhile bought a door, and instructed the panting chairmen on arrival to nail it to the poles, had himself laid carefully on the stretcher, and was borne to Bow.

They were laying out the amputation instruments when a colleague from Bart's arrived and countermanded the operation. The gentleness of the transport, the immobility of the fracture, had left the leg with a sporting chance against amputation, an operation which Pott shuddered was 'terrible to bear and horrible to see'. He escaped infection, which would have been unstoppable and lethal, lay in bed and wrote *On Ruptures*.

Pott was a sociable and prosperous surgeon, his patients enviably including Samuel Johnson and David Garrick. He left the world Pott's disease (deformity of the spine from tuberculous abscess of its bones), Pott's puffy tumour (from infection of the skull), Pott's aneurysm, Pott's gangrene, and chimney-sweep's cancer (from soot encrusting the scrotum, it incited the Chimney Sweeper's Act of 1788, to spare the Water Babies who were pushed up the gentry's fireplaces). He is best remembered for Pott's fracture. This is a fracture-dislocation above the ankle, not the sort Percival Pott suffered at all.

A Colles fracture, which you get from instinctively holding out your arms when you trip over, strikes the radius above the wrist to give the 'dinner-fork' deformity described in 1814 by Abraham Colles (1773–1843) of Dublin. Colles was offered a baronetcy by Lord Melbourne in 1839, but he was so modest that he refused it.

Old Masters

John Abernethy (1764–1831) was a rude surgeon. When he followed Percival Pott at St Bartholomew's, he advised overweight City aldermen, 'Live on sixpence a day, and earn it.' Their overweight wives he counselled, 'Madam, buy a skipping-rope.' Of their constipated corseted daughters: 'Why, madam, do you know there are upwards of thirty yards of bowels squeezed underneath the girdle of your daughters? Go home and cut it, let Nature have fair play, and you will have no need of my advice.'

Abernethy tied off the carotid artery in the neck for bleeding, and the iliac artery inside the belly for aneurysm. Nobody else had dared. Before anaesthesia and antisepsis, the belly was as inviolable as the vaults of the Bank of England. 'He formed an epoch in the history of his profession,' the *Edinburgh Medical Journal* generously complimented a Londoner.

He was a surgeon who hated operating. He was once found by his assistant: 'In the retiring room, after a severe operation, with big tears in his eyes, lamenting the possible failure of what he had just been compelled to do by dire necessity and surgical rule.' He had another weakness. 'I have met with one person who bore evidence to its intoxicating power, such as staggered my own incredulity; for he was a surgeon, and had himself taken opium largely,' de Quincy wrote about John Abernethy in *Confessions of an English Opium-Eater*. He continued by quoting: '"I will maintain," said he, "that I *do* talk nonsense; and, secondly, I will maintain that I do not talk nonsense upon principle, or with any view to profit, but solely and simply," said he – "solely and simply – solely and simply" (repeating it three times over) "because I am drunk with opium; and that daily".'

Everything Abernethy could not operate upon he treated with the ubiquitous mercuric blue pill, which moved the bowels. One Saturday night, he drew aside the daughter who had for weeks nursed a widowed patient: 'I have witnessed your devotion and kindness to your mother. I am in need of a wife, and I think you are the very person that would suit me. My time is incessantly occupied, and I have therefore no leisure for courting. Reflect upon this matter until Monday.' It worked.

Sir Astley Paston Cooper (1768–1841) across the Thames at Guy's, was enthusiastically polite. It made him £15,000 a year, and £600 a year for his butler, who fiddled queue-jumping in the crammed waiting-room. You could then tell a successful surgeon from the line of waiting carriages filling the length of his street. In 1820, Astley Cooper cut a superficial cyst out of George IV's head, and set the going rate for laying knife on King as a baronetcy (Lawrence got the picture). Every morning, Sir Astley conscientiously practised by dissecting corpses for two hours before breakfast (tea and two hot rolls). He was a free-spending fence for the body-snatchers, who demanded at least eight guineas a corpse, which you could get in France for 7s. Sir Astley politely told MPs at a Commons Select Committee on Anatomy in April 1828: 'There is no person, whatever his worldly place, whom I could not dissect if I would.' A contemplation almost as chilling as of losing your seat.

Sir Astley Cooper's rich practice was inherited by Sir Benjamin Collins Brodie (1783–1862), surgeon to St George's Hospital at Hyde Park Corner, at the time it was being rebuilt as the charmingly sited hotel it has since become. Sir Benjamin himself endures as Brodie's abscess (chronic, of the tibia) and Brodie's disease of the breast (big, but benign). In 1858, Sir Benjamin became the first President of the General Medical Council, a body widely assumed to be established for the public disgrace of doctors sexually harassing or horizontalising their patients. The GMC's more consistent use is regulating medical education, so eradicating the medical cowboys who could not attain the official *Register*, the list which confers all necessary doctors' rights from

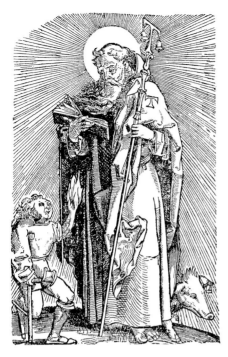

12. *St Anthony and pig, treating patient with St Anthony's Fire.*

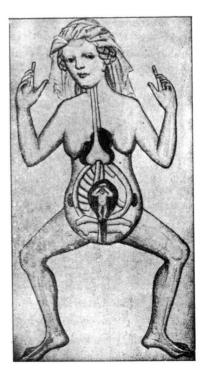

13. *Pregnancy simplified.*

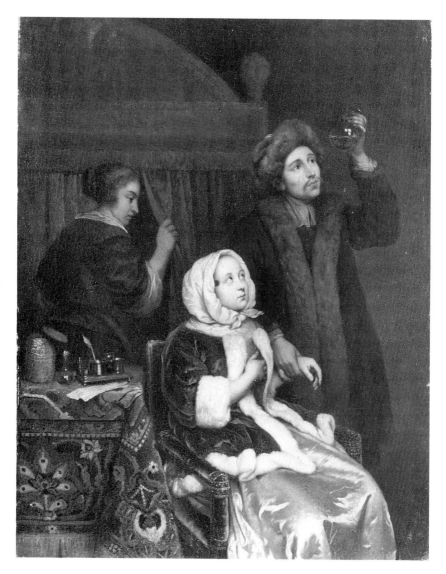

14. *The water of love:* Mal d'Amour *by Gerard Dou.*

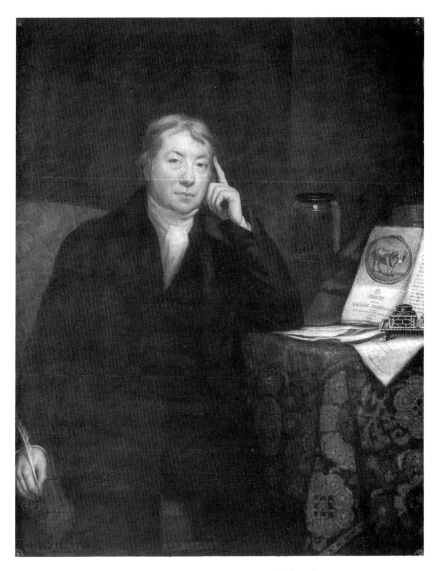

15. *Edward Jenner, the milkmaids' friend.*

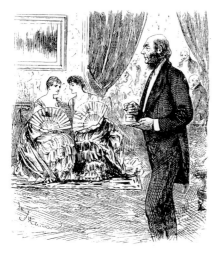

ANNALS OF A WINTER
HEALTH RESORT

Lady Visitor: "OH, THAT'S YOUR DOCTOR, IS IT?
WHAT SORT OF A DOCTOR IS HE?"
Lady Resident: "OH, WELL, I DON'T KNOW MUCH
ABOUT HIS ABILITY; BUT HE'S GOT A VERY
GOOD BEDSIDE MANNER!"

16. Punch *classic.*

Doctor: "WHAT DID YOU OPERATE ON JONES
FOR?"
Surgeon: "A HUNDRED POUNDS."
Doctor: "NO, I MEAN WHAT HAD HE GOT?"
Surgeon: "A HUNDRED POUNDS."

(1925)

17. Punch *chestnut.*

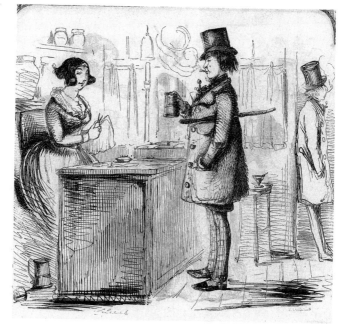

18. Punch *medical student.*

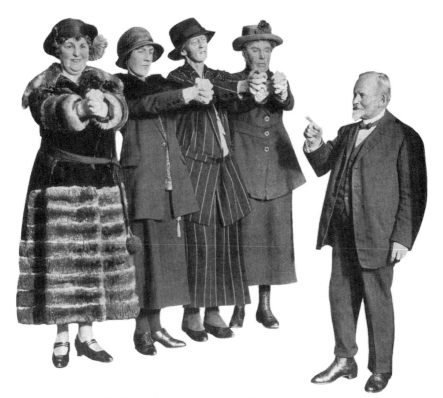

19. *'Every day, in every way . . .' Coué and patients.*

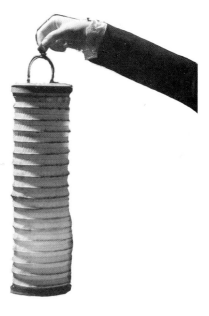

20. *The Lady's lamp (correct version – Florence Nightingale used a Turkish army lamp).*

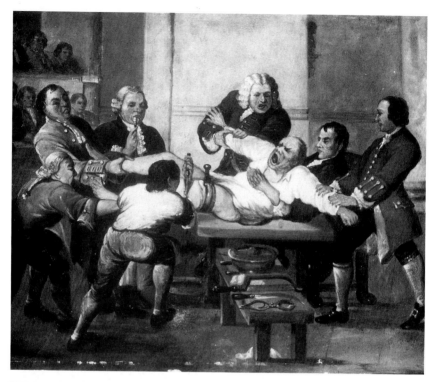

21. *Routine amputation, late eighteenth century.*

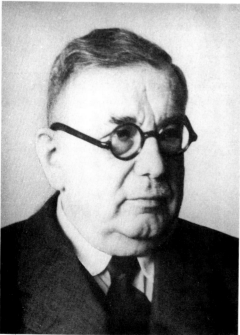

22. *Professor Hörlein of Wuppertal.*

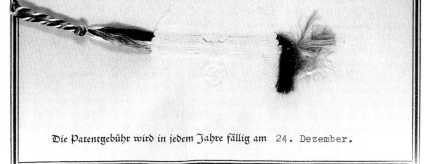

Deutsches Reich

Urkunde
über die Erteilung des Patents

697 297

Für die in der angefügten Patentschrift dargestellte Erfindung ist in dem gesetz-lich vorgeschriebenen Verfahren

dem Dr. Gerhard Domagk in Wuppertal-Elberfeld

ein Patent erteilt worden, welches in der Rolle die oben angegebene Nummer erhalten hat.
Das Patent führt die Bezeichnung

Desinfektions- und Konservierungsmittel

und hat angefangen am   24. Dezember 1933.

Reichspatentamt

Die Patentgebühr wird in jedem Jahre fällig am   24. Dezember.

23. *Sulphonamide patent, 1933: a swastika was overprinted later.*

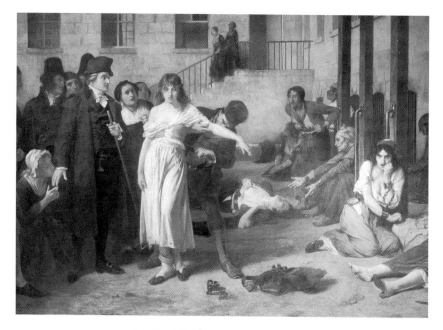

24. *Pinel frees madmen and madwomen.*

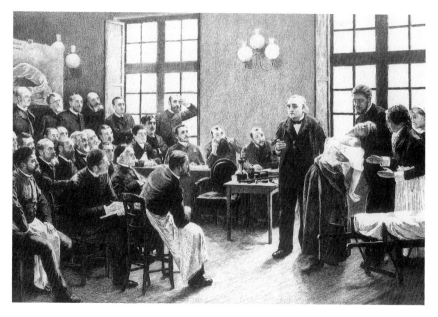

25. *The Charcot show:*
Charcot lecturing on hysteria at the Salpêtrière, Paris.

signing sick-notes to death certificates. Before the GMC, only a third of British doctors had bothered to become qualified.

Across the Solway Firth was James Syme (1799–1870), Lord Lister's father-in-law. He is immortalised by Syme's amputation of the foot. Born in Princes Street, his father a Writer to the Signet, Syme was an essentially Edinburgh man who 'never wasted a word, or a drop of ink, or a drop of blood'. He became Edinburgh's Professor of Surgery by himself pensioning off the incumbent at £300 a year, a canny bargain as his predecessor was then eighty-one. As a student with a penchant for chemistry, Syme noticed that india-rubber dissolved in naphtha rendered cloth waterproof. Had he exploited his discovery, we should all be wearing in rainy weather our symes, not our macintoshes.

Across the Channel, the contracture which draws your fingers into the palm was being treated in 1832 by Baron Guillaume Dupuytren (1777–1835). Dupuytren was the worst sort of surgeon. Vain, contemptuous, overbearing, unscrupulous, he operated *en pantoufles* and repeated irritatingly, if rightly: 'I have been mistaken, but I have been mistaken less than other surgeons.' And as well – utterly infuriatingly – he was a magnificent operator and surpassingly kind to his patients.

Baron Dupuytren's first contracture operation was on a Paris wine-merchant, but the surgeon had stayed his scalpel until he found a dead body with the identical deformity to practise on. The operation persists, the condition is common, its distinguished patients including Mrs Thatcher. It has become suspected of being another of those autoimmune reactions, like rheumatism.

Dupuytren was mean. As a medical student, he took fat from the corpses to light his reading-lamp. When a duchess presented him with a hand-embroidered purse as a tender token of gratitude for saving her life, he snapped that his fee was 5,000 francs. Whereupon, she smilingly removed five 1,000 franc notes from the purse and returned it. She cooed it now contained exactly that, and how modest he was. Dupuytren was 'the brigand of the Hôtel Dieu', who left a fortune. He must once have possessed charm, being supported in youth first by a rich woman from Toulouse and then by a cavalry officer.

Across the Atlantic at Philadelphia, Philip Syng Physick (1768–1837) was the Father of American Surgery. He was an Edinburgh graduate, a pupil of London's John Hunter, and in 1826 he invented the artificial anus. William Wardell Mayo (1819–1911) from Manchester was the father of American surgeons William James (1861–1939) and Charles Horace Mayo (1865–1939), and all three founded the Mayo Clinic in Rochester, Minnesota, the surgical equivalent of the Guggenheim Museum of art on Fifth Avenue.

The Civilising of Surgery

Sir James Paget (1814–99) was a brewer's son, a penniless student, a hack medical journalist, who rose to £10,000 a year and is the only surgeon to make Gilbert and Sullivan. Colonel Calverley sings in *Patience* about the pluck of Lord Nelson on board of the *Victory*, the genius of Bismarck devising a plan, and the 'Coolness of Paget about to trepan'. An honour matching his becoming Serjeant Surgeon to Queen Victoria.

Paget left us Paget's disease of bone (your skull thickens, you have to buy progressively larger hats) and Paget's disease of the nipple (cancer). Paget's voice soared often round the halls of public speaking. 'I divide people into two classes – those who have, and those who have not, heard James Paget,' Mr Gladstone chorused with W. S.

Gilbert. At twenty-nine, Paget became Warden of St Bartholomew's Medical College and married. His bride shivered in the Warden's house at the screams of pre-anaesthetic patients in the operating-theatre next door. 'A chirurgien should have three divers properties in his person. That is to say, a heart as the heart of a lion, his eyes like the eyes of an hawk, and his hands as the hands of a woman,' perceived John Halle (?1529–?1568), surgeon and poet. These qualities were all that the earlier surgeons could bring their patients. They were artists, inspired by anatomy. Now they are interior decorators, creatively rearranging the bodily furniture in the bright lighting of science. The cavities of the body no longer daunt but entice, no tissue cringes secret from the scalpel, organs are transplanted like hardy annuals, microscopical surgery is as unremarkable as television, the surgery of comfort – hips, knees, bunions, varicose veins – rather than the surgery of survival is so everyday that everyone complains bitterly if they do not receive it promptly.

The Stone-cutters

'I will not use the knife, not even, verily, on sufferers from the stone, but I will leave such procedures to the practitioners of the craft,' directed Hippocrates defensively in the Oath.

Stones have been growing in bladders for 7,000 years, evinced by Egyptian mummies. Ancient Arabs and Hindus were cutting for stone, then Celsus and Paracelsus. The sixteenth century had strolling lithotomists like the jugglers and the tinkers. Piere Franco (1505–70), a Huguenot driven from Provence to Lusanne, could nimbly get bladder stones out from above or below (he confessed that failure meant running for your life from the relatives). Frère Jacques de Beaulieu (1651–1719) did it from the side, and gave his fees to the poor. Franciscan Frère Jean de Saint Côme (1703–81) invented a slicker knife, and claimed 90 per cent cures. Newton's and Pope's surgeon, William Cheselden (1688–1752), could do it in a minute, on a good day fifty-four seconds. Many escaped the operation, like Pepys on 7 March 1665: 'Anon I went to make water, not dreaming of anything but my testicle, that by some accident I might have bruised as I used to do – but in pissing, there came from me two stones; I could feel them, and caused my water to be looked into, but without any pain to me in going out.'

In the 1860s, Napoleon III's medical courtiers struggled to hush up an enormous bladder stone, which made the Emperor walk bow-legged, and faint twice in Biarritz after a heavy night with his mistresses. The stone complicated the gonorrheal strictures already up his penis, and prevented his opening the Suez Canal in 1869. The doctors said he had rheumatism, but the Press jeered. Even reporters knew that you did not treat rheumatism with catheters.

The Emperor refused to have a seeking probe pushed up, and commanded his army in the Franco-Prussian War of 1870–71 with towels stuffed down his breeches as nappies. When Napoleon escaped the Third Republic to join the Empress Eugénie outside London, Queen Victoria's surgeons were severer. On 2 and 6 January 1873, the stone was crushed inside Napoleon by urologist Sir Henry Thompson Bt (1820–1904), founder of the Golder's Green crematorium (Millais got the picture), who had performed a royal rehearsal ten years before on Leopold I of Belgium. Joseph Clover gave the chloroform. Everyone was delighted that the Emperor Napoleon's eight-year affliction was finally resolved, but unfortunately three days later the patient died. Such history occurred in the building which is now suburban Chisle-hurst's golf club.

Domestic Science

The year is 1923:

I lay glaring at the ceiling, my forehead covered with drops of cold sweat. I wrung my fingers together lest all sensation should go out of them.

In a while there came three awful moans from the room above and then once more the moving of feet was to be heard, whereby I felt that the operation had begun. I could picture the knife, the great cut, the cold callousness of it all. For what seemed to me to be interminable hours I gazed at the ceiling. Suddenly there was a great commotion in the room above. The table was dragged round rapidly. There were footsteps everywhere. Was the operation over? No. Something had gone wrong. A man dashed downstairs calling for a cab. In a moment I could hear the wheels tear along the street and then return. He had gone to fetch something and rushed upstairs with it . . .

Now, as I gazed upwards, I noticed to my expressionless horror a small round patch of red appear on the white ceiling. I knew it was blood. The spot was as large as a five-shilling piece. It grew until it had become the size of a plate. It became a deeper crimson until at last one awful drop fell upon the white coverlet of my bed. It came down with the weight of lead. I could hardly breathe. Another drop fell with a thud like a stone . . .

Enough!

The heroine of the sanguinary dowsing was a delicate lady in a London nursing-home who was undergoing a rest cure for her nerves, of which it instantly cured her.

Modern surgery is so technical that it must be performed in complex, staff-jostling operating theatres, spiked with monitors and print-outs. These would be impenetrably mysterious to onlookers, did they not appear monotonously on their television. Until the 1930s, major surgery was accomplished in makeshift operating theatres in nursing homes converted from comfortable town houses, or in the houses themselves. Tonsils and even appendices were removed on the kitchen table. Lord Lister operated all over London, his ungainly three-foot-high antiseptic 'donkey engine', undisguised by its cloth, sitting in the brougham leaving his Regent's Park home. Its arrival was eyed by the patient's knowing neighbours with the shudders, jokes and gloating of Tyburn bystanders at the appearance of the hangman with his equipment.

Author of the neurotic lady's horror story was Sir Frederick Treves Bt (1853–1923), who operated on fifty-year-old King Edward VII on 24 June 1902. The King had developed bellyache and was seen by Lord Lister, who diagnosed perityphlitis. This was a vague name for a localised inflamed gut, of which Treves had pioneered the cure by removing the appendix since 1887. In 1889, Charles McBurney (1845–1913) of the Roosevelt Hospital in New York had clarified the condition by targeting the diagnosis on 'McBurney's point', between the umbilicus and the hip, painful in acute appendicitis to the surgeon's finger-tip.

It was all dreadfully inconvenient, because it clashed with the Coronation. This was two days later, which the King suggested could not be postponed as casually as a Sandringham shooting-party. 'Then, Sire, you will go to the Abbey as a corpse,' said the surgeon. The point was taken. The disruption was indeed unthinkable, all those foreign kings and princes already arrived at Victoria Station. Buckingham Palace reeled under problems like, what to be done with the caviar? They kept it on ice, also the 2,500 quails, but the partridge and cutlets had to go to the poor. Crammed hampers were dispatched to charity, and Whitechapel next afternoon enjoyed *consommé de faisan aux quenelles* and *cotelettes de bécassines à la Souvaroff*. The Coronation was postponed to 9 August, and if the caviar kept until then, only the Abyssinian royals stayed to share it.

Edward VII was operated upon at home. He walked to the table and climbed up, Queen Alexander took his hand, retained it into anaesthesia and resumed before he was conscious. The Royal patient saved innumerable lives from the vague perityphlitis diagnosis, by giving Treves' operation the *éclat* which his descendants brought to polo.

Treves was no courtier, in bed at 10 pm to be up at 6 for writing. He was a friend of Thomas Hardy, he held a master mariner's certificate, and could have captained the Royal yacht as well. Appropriately for a surgeon, Treves was an incisive and astringent author. His story of the Elephant Man, whom he befriended at the London Hospital, became a West End and Broadway hit, though unfortunately by then Treves was both dead and out of copyright.

Putting on a Brave Face

Plastic surgery's 2,000-year old origin was adultery in India. This was taken by Hindus with a seriousness requiring the matrimonial intruder's nose to be cut off. The facial and social blemish could be repaired by skin from the cheek or forehead, fashioned by a pattern cut on a leaf, and stitched over the hole. The operation was improved in Bologna in 1597 by Gasparo Tagliacozzi (1546–99), who raised a skin flap from the arm, bound the arm to the nose, and when the transplant took to its new bed he cut the arm free at its roots. They had been doing it amateurishly in Sicily for a century: Branca of Catanea was the 'man of great abilities, who had learned the art of restoring a nose, either by supplying it from the arm of the patient, or by infixing upon the part the nose of a slave'.

The Church objected so angrily to Tagliacozzi's improving God's handiwork, they dug him up from a convent grave and replaced him in unconsecrated earth. All this got nose-jobs a bad name. In 1788, facial plastic surgery was banned in Paris, as wicked.

Johann Friedrich Dieffenbach (1792–1847), a former Mecklenberg cavalryman, cut the eye muscles to cure squint (successfully) and the tongue muscles to cure stammering (unsuccessfully). At the Charité Hospital in Berlin, he began reconstructing faces affected by trauma or tumour and reuniting cleft palates. Bereft of anaesthesia, the patient was sat facing a window, an assistant grasping his head, and was told to take deep breaths, with mouthwash and pause for gasps offered between incisions. Dieffenbach was a friend of Heine and of King Wilhelm IV of Prussia, who often used to look in at his operations, bringing his family.

In London, Sir William Fergusson (1808–77) operated, mostly successfully, on 134 cleft palates and 400 hare lips. He had been obliged to emigrate from Edinburgh, where James Syme was not wasting a drop of the going private practice. Sir William believed it was 'a grand thing when by prescience even the tip of a thumb can be saved'. This was merciful conservatism when amputation was practised with the enthusiasm of Alice's Queen of Hearts. Sir William was also a virtuoso violinist and lithotomist: 'Look out sharp,' said one of the audience, 'because if you only wink, you'll miss the operation altogether.'

Modern plastic surgery was a by-product of gunpowder. It was conceived in 1917 by an artistically-inclined surgeon, Sir Harold Delf Gillies (1882–1960), in the ugly London suburb of Sidcup, at the brand-new Queen's Hospital, which now breasts the passage from the Blackwall Tunnel to the Channel Tunnel.

'A beautiful woman is worth preserving and should be kept youthful while she is still young enough to enjoy it,' Harold Gillies in 1957 corrected Paris of 1788 and God her Maker. Gillies was a New Zealander, a throat surgeon, a descendant of Edward (*Book of Nonsense*) Lear, an RAMC captain in 1915. A jaw surgeon at the American Hospital in Paris had lent him a textbook just arrived from Germany: 'It being a rather informal war, the enemy did not seem to mind our learning of the good work they were doing on jaw fractures and wounds about the mouth.' Thus the textbook's author, Lindemann, inaugurated through Gillies a specialty which improved the morale of British and American forces in two wars against his own country.

Top British surgical brass was Sir Arbuthnot (colon specialist) Lane, who encouraged Gillies at Sidcup. Gillies was joined there by a surgically-inclined artist, Henry Tonks (1862–1937), once Sir Frederick Treves' house-surgeon at the London Hospital. In 1917, Tonks was Professor at the Slade School of Fine Arts, the instructor of Augustus John and William Orpen, but he had become a fellow of the Royal College of Surgeons in 1888, and now rejoined his old profession in the RAMC. Tonks drew the wounds, the repairs and the results, and surely improved Gillies' artistry in skin grafts, skin flaps, and skin pedicles like Tagliacozzi's.

Eccentric, cantankerous, egotist, expert at golf and angling, Gillies was outshone in World War Two by another New Zealander, his cousin, the glittering and autocratic Sir Archibald Hector McIndoe (1910–60), with his 'Guinea Pig Club' of RAF patients at East Grinstead south of London. Perhaps the repeated operations necessary on these patients' faces justified their often imperfect results; perhaps plastic surgeons' less sensational work on burns and hands was worthier. But a young man in a Spitfire was encouraged to know that there were clever surgeons waiting to repair his terrifying mutilation.

Between the wars plastic surgery had grown, after them it flourished. New faces, new noses, no trouble (McIndoe's delicately tipped-up noses were instantly recognisable across footlights or dinner-tables). Women became so fussy about their breasts that bosoms could be commanded in sizes like bras. 'Often while lifting a face I have had a feeling of guilt that I am merely making money. Yet is it not justified if it brings even a little extra happiness to a soul who needs it?' Gillies encouraged himself. Perhaps the happiness is transient, and the melancholy resentment which is targeted on your own features is transferred to something, or to someone, else.

Headline Surgery

On 3 December 1967, at Groote Schuur Hospital in Cape Town, Professor Christiaan Neethling Barnard (b 1922) performed the first heart transplant operation, so combining natural, human and emotional forces of Shakespearian intensity. On 25 November 1974, he bettered it by performing the first double-heart transplant. The idea was not new. It had occurred to John Hunter two centuries earlier in London, where a human tooth which he transplanted into a cock's comb is viewable in the Royal College of Surgeons.

Our dead body is like a curate's egg, parts of it are excellent. But the healthy bits cannot readily replace others' sick ones, because the body roughly rejects immunological gate-crashers. On 23 December 1954, at Peter Brent Brigham Hospital in Boston, a healthy kidney was transplanted from one brother (you need only one kidney) into another with two dud ones, and afforded him another nine years of life. But these brothers were identical twins. The transplant trick is matching donors' and recipients' tissues, then using the new immunosuppressive drugs which can artificially make identical twins of us all. These drugs quell the unfriendly welcome until the new host gets used to the visitor, thence they rub along happily together. Kidneys, lungs, hearts and livers are now exchanged by living and dead human beings with the benevolence of Christmas presents.

The incoming kidney is not placed in the loin but tucked more conveniently into the pelvis. The 'harvesting' is grotesque even to seasoned doctors. The transplant surgeon, summoned urgently by an unsleeping organisation, thoughtfully explains to the local staff that this is not to be an episode of conventional surgery. The anaesthetist wheels in the subject – pink, warm, breathing regularly through the action of a mechanical respirator, heart beating, but dead. The surgeon forthwith makes an incision of post-mortem room generosity, removes heart, lungs, kidneys, liver and, while he is at it, other useful bits like pancreas or an adrenal gland. These are put on ice for dramatic transport by helicopter or amid flashing blue lights to their selected recipients, who have already been summoned with their suitcases to their nearest transplant hospitals. The anaesthetist switches off the breathing machine. The subject turns ashen and cold, and unexpectedly sweats. The corpse is taken to the mortuary and the operating team drink their coffee thoughtfully.

Lest I incur from this description the shame of a single torn-up donor card – a stupid television programme once had them ripped by handfuls – please believe me that the subject is already dead beyond recall. 'Brain dead' is pronounced only after tests which sound the lowermost functions of life and win no response. A donor card is a remarkable possession. Any human who suffers tragic injury or brain haemorrhage can with Biblical sublimity by his death give life.

The Historical Achievement of Both Medicine and Surgery

Good, but limited. Ashes to ashes, dust to dust, if the cancer don't get us the arteriosclerosis must.

SEVEN

Sex and its Snags

All the world loves loving, but it entails the bothersome inconveniences of pregnancy and disease.

The Pain of Sex

The history of contraception is drearily predictable. It started jollily enough, with Boswell. The man whom Johnson found very clubable was also very clapable. James Boswell suffered nineteen attacks of gonorrhea, starting before his first meeting Johnson in 1763 aged twenty-two, and ending in 1795, when he was carried home from a Literary Club dinner with acute retention of urine, and shortly succumbed to thirty-five years' overuse of the waterworks. Boswell had also twelve children, of whom five were illegitimate. The only effective treatment of gonorrhea was applicable to the strictures, which developed below the bladder after the infective 'gleet'. This was 'sounding', by the passage up the penis of curved metal rods, which Boswell hated to the point of fainting. Another literary figure entertaining such a dislike was Thackeray.

Boswell was a condom crusader. He could buy them conveniently in Leicester Square at the sign of the Rising Sun, condoms designed for gentlemen, of sheep's or goat's gut, pickled, scented, eight inches long, delicately fashioned on glass moulds by the hands of the proprietress, Mrs Phillips. Her best quality 'Baudruches Superfines' were secured round the neck with ribbon, which could be in regimental colours. (They are viewable, carelessly tossed on the floorboards with the oystershells and chicken-bones and stays in Hogarth's *Rake's Progress* of 1736.)

It is sad that the Englishman's obsession with club ties is so unthoughtfully still not thus indulged. The rich blue and crimson of the Brigade of Guards, the sunshine and tomato of MCC, the salmon and cucumber of the Garrick Club, would insert artistic embellishment into an inescapably inelegant performance. For Mrs Phillips's more cautious customers, her 'Superfine Double' was tailored of two superimposed and gummed caecums, the blind end of the sheep's bigger gut. Such prophylactic ovine tripe was first advertised as 'An Engine for the Prevention of Harms by Love-Adventures', in *The Tatler* of 12 May 1709.

Boswell did not *like* condoms. 'Armour' numbed the fun with the Lizzies, Nannies, Louisas, Megs, into whom he lovingly adventured all over London, whether in the taverns of Covent Garden and the Strand, accomplishing sixpenny knee-tremblers in St James's Park and on Westminster Bridge, or with seventeen-year-old Alice Briggs in the garden of No 10 Downing Street (before it was official property). Boswell preferred the linen sort, which needed wetting first (he dipped them in the Hyde Park Canal). They were more economical than Mrs Phillips's Baudruches, because you could take them to the condom laundrette in St Martin's Lane, run by Jenny. Boswell was a poor public health advertisement for condoms, but only from the non-unique inconvenience of never seeming to have one on him when he wanted it.

The current coffee-house jingle for condoms extolled their protection against 'the ills of Shankers, or Cordee, or Buboes Dire!' But it mentioned the secondary avoidance of 'the Big Belly and the Squalling Brat', wherein lay future trouble.

Avoiding the Issue

Separating human enthusiasm for sexual bliss from human reproduction causes majestic fuss. The Roman Catholic Church is reasonably concerned with the sanctity of human life, but equally to express its authority by meddling with fundamental bodily functions. Holding the congregation by the testicles is a more effective extractor of loyalty than making them eat fish on Friday. Alternative natural contraception by menstrual rhythm, prolonged breast-feeding, and coitus interruptus may be religiously blameless, but is copulatory Russian roulette.

In 1798, the Rev Thomas Robert Malthus (1766–1834) indicated that a world continuing copulating at its present rate would be a world eventually dying through self-inflicted starvation. The only cheerful items he could discern to cause delay were unwholesome occupations, severe labour, extreme poverty, bad nursing, large towns, excesses, diseases, epidemics, wars and famines. The genial Malthus (father of three) was not a malthusian. He refuted contraception, recommending instead that the world saved its bacon by moral restraint, to be encouraged by raising the age of consent to marriage. This was an absurdly optimistic remedy to a grim menace. Equally rational people saw mechanical, rather than moral, restraint as more attractively workable. This caused outrage.

The Solicitor-General was saying on behalf of the affronted at the Guildhall in the summer of 1877:

> I say this is a dirty, filthy book, and the test of it is that no human being would allow that book to lie on his table; no decently educated English husband would allow even his wife to have it. The object of it is to enable persons to have sexual intercourse, and not to have that which in the order of Providence is the natural result of that sexual intercourse.

The title was *Fruits of Philosophy, or the Private Companion of Young Married People*, by American Dr Charles Knowlton (1800–50). It had been published (illustrated) the year before in Bristol by Henry Cook, who got two years hard labour. In present trouble were Charles Bradlaugh (1833–91), ex-errand-boy and ex-trooper, a truly independent MP who refused to swear on the Parliamentary Bible, was ejected from the House by the Sergeant-at-Arms, and locked up under Big Ben for two days (surely, sleep impossible). He was four times unseated by Parliament and five times elected by the persistently sensible shoemaking town of Northampton, until Parliament got fed up, and he represented them unto death.

And Anne Besant (1847–1933), separated from her vicar husband, later a Theosophist, who discovered the new Messiah (Jeddu Krishnamurti of Madras, aged fourteen, she adopted him and paraded him round the world from 1910 to 1925, he used regularly to step out of his body during sleep). With Bradlaugh, she had formed the Freethought Publishing Company deliberately to republish *Fruits of Philosophy*.

They both got six months and a £200 fine, which was quashed on appeal, but only technically, through a verbal fault in the indictment. The judges warned that if reoffending they would be for it. Bradlaugh sold the confiscated copies stamped in red RECOVERED FROM THE POLICE, a stroke of sound publishing, and Anne Besant's 1877 paperback *The Law of Population* sold 175,000. When a Leeds dermatologist, Henry Arthur Allbutt (1846–1904), published his sixpenny *The Wife's Handbook* in 1886, the General Medical Council struck him from the medical *Register* for unprofessional conduct, but he was compensated by the book's doing half a million.

The Guildhall of 1877 echoed in the Old Bailey of 1960. Buzfuzed Attorney-General Mervyn Griffith-Jones:

> The book abounds in bawdy conversation. The word 'copulate' or 'copulation' occurs no less than thirty times. I have added them up, but I do not guarantee that I have added them all up. 'Vulva' fourteen times; 'testicles' thirteen times; 'faeces' and 'anus' six times apiece; 'penis' four times; 'urination' three times, and so on.

He gave point to this ludicrous catalogue by using not my technical words, but the common ones he might himself use for them at weekends. It was the trial of *Lady Chatterly's Lover*, which attracted the Attorney-General's charming concern that one's servant might read it – in an era when the cheap tweeny was being replaced by the cheaper twin-tub.

Morals are largely an expression of history and geography. Anything goes, but not everywhere. Hindus are allowed no drink but numerous wives, Christians can get drunk as often as we like but are bound, as Saki puts it, to 'the Western custom of one wife and hardly any mistresses'. It was wicked in the USA to toast Washington's birthday in 1933, but patriotic in 1934. In Fiji in the 1830s, even cannibalism was socially acceptable, with the donor's brains saved as a treat for the ladies.

'But there are two moralities,' indicated Flaubert. 'One is petty and conventional; it is the invention of men and changes endlessly, a congeries of prosaic and clamorous nothings, which makes as much noise as the imbeciles down there. But the other lives in that eternity which is all round and all above us, like the fields and the woods and the blue sky spreading its radiance on our earth.'

The morality which is as inconsequential as that imbecillic chatter from Flaubert's Agricultural Show is appealing. It so readily incites solicitous condemnation of its everyday infringements, when performed by other people.

The Condom Comes into its Own

The vulcanisation of rubber in 1843 did miracles for the condom, as for golf-balls. By the 1920s, condoms were constructed with the reassuringly stout reliability of tyres for the Daimler. They formed mildly shameful pocket-contents, like cigarettes today. They were stocked invisibly by raffish chemists, involving lingering – reading the labels on Sanatogen and Parrish's Food and Zam-Buck – until the other customers had left. Condoms were more fearlessly and fittingly preserved for society by their distribution through the surgeons' ancestors, the barbers ('And anything for the person, sir?'), which accounted for the male fashion earlier this century of extremely short hair.

Our Florence Nightingale of the marriage-bed was Marie Charlotte Carmichael Stopes (1880–1959), whom God addressed personally in 1920 amid her yews at Leatherhead. Her *Married Love* sold 1,000 copies a week. Its incidental suggestion, that the wife should clamp the husband in her legs during love, invoked the criticism of an Australian MP: 'Let us in the name of true, normal manhood and womanhood, and indeed in the name of the British Empire, endeavour to keep the imagination down at all costs.'

Marie Stopes was PhD Munich, and her first marriage, in Montreal to an American botanist, was annulled in 1916 because after five years she persisted as *virgo intacta*. Backed worthily by Arnold Bennett, H. G. Wells and contralto Dame Clara Butt, Marie Stopes opened in 1921 a Mothers' Clinic in Islington, where they inserted rubber pessaries into the working class. All ended in libellous tears. The Archbishop of Westminster, Cardinal Bourne, himself gave £400 towards the £10,000 Catholic fund backing their championed defendant, Dr Halliday Gibson Sutherland (1882–1960), who explained: 'The ordinary decent instincts of the poor are against these practices . . . the poor are the natural victims of those who seek to make experiments on their fellows.'

It's the poor wot gets the blame. This was a valuable time in the history of contraception for it to receive the application of Marie Stopes' insufferable egoism and earnestness.

Condoms were named after Dr or possibly Colonel Condom, who was an Englishman or perhaps a Frenchman, and perhaps a courtier of Charles II, or maybe never existed at all. The best a Latin dictionary can do is *condo*, 'to put in, to thrust', also to bottle fruit. The nearest the Oxford Dictionary gets is condoma, which is a striped antelope with spiral horns. Condom (pop. 6,781) between Bordeaux and Toulouse is prouder of its armagnac, though Bishop Bossuet of its Cathédrale St-Pierre in 1669 was summoned to Paris by Louis XIV to instruct the young Dauphin in French letters.

Nobody used to call them condoms. The unpoetical Americans flooded into World War Two with rubbers, while the British made fidgety precoital jokes about 'Free love with a capital F L'. The word entered respectable conversation only in the years of Mrs Thatcher, along with 'money'. The condom now rises supremely again as sanitary wear. Its shamefaced opponents can hardly bleat about the sanctity of human life, when condomless copulation can extinguish this wholesale with AIDS. There is even a 'Femidom', resembling a bin-liner.

A Matter of Life and Birth

The dispersion of the pill in the mid-twentieth century was an equivalent liberator of women to that of the mangle in the mid-nineteenth. All that reliable female contraception now demands is a memory efficient and sober enough to swallow it. Even this is superfluous with the 'morning after' pill. But such an afterthought stirs ethical excitement, through upsetting the *status quo* rather than preventing it. A post-coital pill resembles an abortion, which ignites righteous wrath, to the pitch of respectable people marching through the streets with banners, and the shaming of MPs with intrauterine photographs of embryos seemingly sucking their thumbs, a habit which they are happily free from.

Regnier de Graaf (1641–73) discovered conception. This Dutch anatomist is memorialised in the Graafian follicle, the bumps on the surface of the two ovaries, which cup the unfertilised eggs. Everybody had previously agreed with Aristotle that the sperm did it all alone. Before that, it took a surprising time before mankind grasped the protracted sexual connection.

Abortion is as old as conception. On 18 July 1938, Aleck William Bourne (1886–1974), son of a Wesleyan minister, a London consultant gynaecologist of crystalline respectability and austere personality, was indicted at the Old Bailey for using an instrument to procure a miscarriage. Top penalty was penal servitude for life. It was all in the Offences Against the Person Act of 1861, Section 58. But the judge unfolded that abortion was an offence under English common law, even before Parliament existed. Hippocrates too was against it: 'I will not give to a woman a pessary to cause abortion,' his Oath bound doctors. This promise has become fenestrated like the succeeding one: 'I will keep pure and holy my life and my art.'

On 14 June, at 10 o'clock in the morning, Bourne had aborted at St Mary's Hospital in Paddington a fourteen-year-old girl, who was six weeks pregnant, having been raped twice while held down by five off-duty Lifeguards, after being invited to inspect a mare with a green tail in a horse-box at Horse Guards Parade, Whitehall. She had earlier been turned down at St Thomas's Hospital across the river, on the grounds that the foetus might be a future prime minister. The girl's bewildered parents were so respectable that they knew of no traditional old women in back streets with knitting-needles. Three years earlier, Bourne had done the same disencumberance for a girl of fifteen. His house-surgeon had prudently quit the operating-theatre, refusing to assist an illegal operation. This time, Bourne had told the Attorney-General that he was going to. At the end of his operating-list that evening, detectives arrived at the hospital to remove him to Paddington police-station.

Bourne's liberty balanced at the Old Bailey on the danger to the juvenile mother's life, presented by his counsel as a reasonable excuse. Was her life endangered if her health was endangered? Would it be endangered by lifelong wretchedness? If you are preserving her life, you must presumably equally preserve her health, otherwise, who knows, she might drop dead? 'It is an issue that has never before been raised,' said the judge uncomfortably. Or was the suspicion justified, of Bourne flamboyantly flouting the law to change the law?

Everyone leant backwards over bench, bar, and jury-box to acquit, which ten men and two women performed in forty minutes after a two-day trial. It was the glorification of common sense, a quality undeservedly uneulogised by poets. The verdict set going sensible notions on abortion which were legalised in 1967, despite the most profound principles, prejudices, prudery and pompousness. The only blemish to the comforting story is the suspicion of its heroine being a 'half-crown girl', hanging round the Horse Guards on duty.

The circumstances of the Bourne case recurred in Dublin, when a fourteen-year-old girl, who was raped, went to London for an abortion but obediently returned home after the Irish Attorney-General obtained an injunction to stop her. The date was February, 1992. Irish outcry had the judgement reversed.

In South America, the commonest cause of death in women under fifty is illegal abortion.

The philosopher who 'Round him much embryo, much abortion lay', faces an undignified, persistent muddle about the sacred moment when life begins. When does the infant lead a separate existence, before it is so obviously mewling and puking in the midwife's arms? The moment of joyous union between sperm and egg is inappropriate, because so many, like matrimonial unions, fail to last. In Britain, we wisely left it to the House of Lords. Their Lordships decided with the Human Fertilization and Embryology Bill to create human life at the twenty-fourth week after successful sex, performing on 18 October 1990 what God did on the sixth day.

Couples who conceive children they do not want are mirrored by couples who want children but cannot conceive. The plight of these second unfortunates has been attended by gynaecologists with less extraneous fuss. Bossy persons object more to others doing what they think they should not, rather than dubiously achieving what they think they should.

A Pox Upon Us

In 1492, Columbus discovered America. After his return in 1493, the Old World discovered a new disease. It was despondently catalogued by Nicolo Leoniceno (1428–1524), Professor of Physic at Ferrara: painful pustules on the private parts spreading to the body and face, rashes, ulcers, buboes, black pustules, carbuncles, agonising and swollen joints, lassitude, fever, rotting flesh, blindness and death, the symptoms lingering for years in survivors. Giovanni di Vigo (1460–1520), who was the Vatican surgeon while Michelangelo was doing the decorating, in 1514 wrote a best-selling textbook *Practica in Arte Chirurgica Copiosa* (fifty-two editions), which imparted: 'This disease is contagious, chiefly if it chance through copulation of a man with an unclean woman.'

This connection had previously been doubted, because 'it infected those which were religious.'

Hieronymus Frascastorius of Verona, envisager of the infective fomite, in 1530 wrote in a long Virgilian poem:

He first wore Buboes dreadful to the sight,
First felt strange Pains and sleepless past the Night:
From him the Malady receiv'd its name,

The neighbouring Shepherds catcht the spreading Flame:
At last in City and in Court 'twas known,
And seiz'd the ambitious Monarch on his throne.

The poem's hero was:

> A shepherd once (distrust not ancient Fame)
> Possest these Downs, and *Syphilus* his Name.
> A thousand Heifers in these Vales he fed.
> A thousand Ews to those fair Rivers led . . .

(The translation is by our Poet Laureate of 1692, Nahum Tate, who did also 'While Shepherds Watched their Flocks by Night'.)

So syphilis became the shuddering eponym of four centuries. Frascastorius had called his poem *Of the French Disease*. Giovanni Di Vigo had earlier noticed in his textbook: 'The Frenchmen call it the disease of Naples, because the soldiers brought it from hence into France. The Neapolitans call it the French disease, for it appeared first when they came to Naples, and so other languages call it by other names.' In this outburst of infected nationalism, it was the Polish disease to the Germans and the German disease to the Poles and the French disease to the Spaniards and the Turkish disease to everyone vague on geography (the British predictably sided with the Spanish and Neapolitans). Nobody thought of blaming the Haitians and Cubans, who had provided Columbus's crew with the traditional entertainment for Jack ashore.

'There often follows this foul sin the foul disease, now called by us the pox,' said Mr Wiseman in *Mr Badman*. 'A disease so nauseous and stinking, so infectious to the whole body, and so entailed to this sin, that hardly are any common with unclean women, that they have more or less a touch of it to their shame.'

If you smoke, you may get cancer of the lung from the smoke. If you drink, you may get cirrhosis of the liver from the alcohol. If you are sexy, you may catch a sexually transmitted disease, as you might catch influenza from being social. To welcome this infection as a punishment holily fitting the crime – as so many have agreed with Bunyan since 1680 – is a merciless expression of sanctimonious nonsense.

The difficult French surgeon Baron Dupuytren had a more charitable approach: 'Have you been with prostitutes?' 'No, how could you even think of it?' the patient replied. 'Then they have been with you,' said Dupuytren.

Syphilis later flourished less fearsomely. It budded with a chancre, blossomed into a rich red rash, then lay dormant in forgetfulness until in the autumn of life, when it sprouted aneurysms, caused staggering and stumbling, and brought madness with delusions of grandeur, also noticeable oddities in the offshoots. A students' *aide-mémoire*:

> There was a young man of Herne Bay
> Who thought that the syph went away.
> Now he's got tabes
> And bandy-legged babies
> And thinks he's the Queen of the May.

Keeping it in the Family

Many historical figures and men of importance have been thought syphilitic. This may be through delusions of grandeur occurring in them naturally. Henry VIII was suspected through a string of stillborn or sickly babies – syphilis is conveyed through the mother, presumably infected by the father – and by his ulcers, bone sinuses and general behaviour. It is ironic to condemn Oscar

Wilde to a syphilitic death. He died from an abscess of the brain spreading from an infected ear, which had augmented the misery of Reading Gaol. Oscar's father Sir William Wilde (1815–76) of Dublin was a pioneer ear specialist, the able author of *Aural Surgery* (also of *The Narrative of a Voyage to Madeira*), and the creator of Wilde's incision for the ear-infected mastoid bone in the skull. Bustling Sir William treated the poor from a disused Dublin stable, was Commissioner for the Irish Census, and discovered prehistoric dwellings in the bogs. He wrote of ear infection: 'We can never tell how, when, or where it will end.' When it ended for his son, with the necessity of an expensive operation in 1900 in Paris, Oscar sighed: 'Ah, well, then, I suppose I shall have to die beyond my means.'

The descendants of Sir Winston Churchill fuss over his father Lord Randolph ('Randy Pandy') Churchill being assumed syphilitic. The accusation lies in the 1925 biography of the awful Frank Harris, who according to Oscar Wilde 'has been received in all the great houses – once'. Harris recounted that Lord Randolph, dining as an Oxford undergraduate with Jowett at Balliol in 1869, felt a tickling in the trousers. He anxiously asked a footman for the lavatory: 'Yes! There was a little, round, very red pimple.' After a drunken evening at the Bullingdon Club, Randy Pandy had reportedly woken in a filthy bedroom beside a dirty old woman with grey hair and one long yellow tooth in her top jaw that waggled as she said: 'Oh, lovie, you're not going to leave me?' (Frank Harris was an equally renowned *littérateur* and *menteur*.)

In the summer of 1893, after he had been Secretary for India and Chancellor of the Exchequer, Lord Randolph consulted his Grosvenor Square physician with speech difficulty, tongue tremor, a numb left arm, staggering, violence, apathy, delusions and confusion, and was reasonably diagnosed as suffering from advanced syphilis.

But syphilis is a shadowy assassin and an agile mimic. Queen Victoria's physician Sir William Gull cautioned his students: 'However clever you are, you are sure to overlook phthisis, syphilis, and itch' (scabies).

It was impossible to tell certainly who had syphilis or not before 1906, when August von Wassermann (1866–1925) of Berlin invented his handy blood test, the famous 'Wasserman reaction'. The *Treponema pallidum*, the thin, spiral microbe, corkscrewing its way through the body and causing all the trouble, had been discovered in Hamburg in 1906 by an innkeeper's son, the zoologist Fritz Richard Schaudinn (1871–1906). This was another expression of the German genius at the time for discovering new microbes, as that of the British for discovering new colonies.

The treatment of syphilis had stayed unvaried since Giovanni di Vigo. It was succinctly put: 'A night of Venus and a lifetime of Mercury'. The mercury was either slapped on or swallowed, both administrations diluted with hope. The only public health measure against syphilis was the German suppression of mixed bathing.

Mercury was ousted by arsenic with Ehrlich's 606 injection in 1909, but this vastly improved treatment was still limited and hazardous. By 1942, the *Treponema Pallidum* (like the gonococcus that had so bothered Boswell) was found susceptible to penicillin. On 26 June 1944, three weeks after D-Day, America expressed repayment of Columbus' microbial invasion of Europe by officially adopting penicillin, then pouring from American drug factories, as the routine treatment of syphilis for the United States Army.

'There are only two diseases I can certainly cure, gout and syphilis,' cheerfully declared a London physician whom I consulted for one of them. In the Pall Mall gentlemen's clubs of the eighteenth century he would have been a beloved and busy doctor.

The Interesting History of Obstetrics and Gynaecology

There is none. Women who joyfully accepted the Victorian Solicitor-General's recommendation – to have that which in the order of Providence is the natural result of sexual intercourse – were traditionally attended by midwives. These were instructed by *The Byrth of Mankynde*, translated (via Latin) by Thomas Raynalde (*c* 1540) from the German of Eucharius Röslin's (*c* 1513) *Rosengarten*, which was the only update for fourteen centuries of a Roman obstetrical treatise by the memorably named Soranus (AD 78–117). From the *Rosengarten* pictures, the mother sat beside her four-poster amid her relatives and midwives, skirted to the ankles, groaning on a birth stool, tub and ewer waiting to wash the baby, while the attendant astrologer looked through the window and cast the foetus's horoscope.

In the eighteenth century was born the man-midwife, who was equally unpopular among his fellow surgeons (pride) and with the midwives (jealousy).

'A great horse godmother of a he-midwife,' a midwife of Haymarket called Tobias Smollett's friend William Smellie (1697–1763) of Pall Mall. Smellie was an exponent of the obstetrical forceps, the *tire-tête* conceived by Peter Chamberlen (1560–1631). Chamberlen was a Huguenot fled from Paris, doing well enough in London to attend Charles I's Queen Henrietta Maria after she aborted in 1628, when the midwife had fainted from fright. The Chamberlens were a medical family (they delivered Queen Anne in 1692), who kept the secret of the forceps for 125 years. A descendant sold it in 1693 to

a Dutchman, who was the son of Hendrik van Roon-
huyze (1625–?), the master of Caesarean section. Smellie
clothed his forceps blades with leather, to spare the
mother the chilling clink of interlocking steel as he set
to work. He taught a thousand students to use them, by
delivering a leather baby-doll installed head-first into the
bony basin of a female skeleton's pelvis, at three guineas
a time.

Gynaecology was invented by the Americans. It originated in the South, to repair the ravages of obstetrics out
in the sticks, mostly upon slaves. The ovary was first
removed in December 1809 (no anaesthetics) in Ken-
tucky, by Ephraim McDowell (1771–1830), who had
studied in Edinburgh. The patient was farmer's wife Mrs
Jane Todd Crawford, who suffered an ovarian cyst, travelled sixty miles on horseback from log cabin to operation, was aged forty-seven and lived to be seventy-eight.

Handsome James Marion Sims (1813–83) of Alabama
designed Sims position (flopping forward on the left side,
right thigh drawn up, left arm dangling behind the back,
it occurred to him when examining a woman thrown
from a horse) and Sims vaginal speculum (adapted from
a bent spoon), which together could see into a woman 'as
no man had ever seen it before'. Marion Sims invented
the operation to repair the leaking fistula which developed between bladder and vagina, which he brought to
Europe in 1861, when he was avoiding the Civil War. He
performed it before Napoleon's veteran Baron Larrey, and
immediately extended his practice from the Hudson to
the Elbe. Sims had moved to New York to found the
Hospital for Women in 1855, his statue is viewable in
Bryant Park, on 42nd Street behind the Public Library.

Gynaecology, like surgery, had its fashions. The uterus
was as darkly suspected of floating as the kidney, and
was surgically, according to Sir Clifford Allbutt, 'impaled
on a stem or perched on a twig'. Rubber pessaries shaped

like horse-collars were inserted vaginally for pelvic pain and to stop the uterus falling out. Hysterectomy and clitoridectomy were inflicted in the 1900s as freely as Sir Arbuthnot Lanes' colectomies. Gynaecology surprises in being a predominantly male specialty. I once asked a gynaecologist who was immensely able, honoured and rich, what fascinating conclusions a lifetime had brought about women. He thought deeply, and said: 'Woman is a constipated biped with pain in the back.'

EIGHT

Dead Ends

Among the greatest discoveries of medicine are the generally belated ones that some treatments are utterly useless.

Colon, Full Stop

People do so fuss about their sex lives and their bowels. Sir 'Willie' Arbuthnot Lane Bt (1856–1943), of Guy's Hospital in London, became the exculpatory genius of the bowels, as Professor Sigmund Freud (1859–1939) of Vienna delightfully became of sex.

The colon is a tube 7.5 centimetres wide and 1.5 metres long, taking over the guts at the appendix. It ascends to the ribs and sags across to the left flank, before descending again to the rectum and the open air. It has an absorbent lining and a muscular wall to push things along. Its contents are the residues of food digested by the body's chemicals, bile, and lots of mostly innocuous bacteria. This mixture is slimy and smelly, but not sensationally more evil than dandruff.

The velvety lining of the colon absorbs water and drugs. Before intravenous drips became safe and effective during World War Two, the necessary replacement fluids for a sick body were given through the colon. It was fashionable then to administer wasting patients nutrient enemas, some impressively complicated, a mixed grill per rectum.

The shadowy menace of the colon had been lurking since the fourteenth century, when 'clyster' entered the fundament and the language. By 1622, Massinger and Decker were rudely calling the doctor 'Thou stinking clyster-pipe'. But by the next century, clystering enjoyed a popularity among the fastidious of dieting today.

Pope was writing fashionably in *The Dunciad* in 1728:

> In office here fair Cloacina stands,
> And ministers to Jove with purest hands . . .
> She oft had favoured him, and favours yet.
> Renewed by ordure's sympathetic force
> As oiled with magic juices for the course,
> Vigorous he rises; from the effluvia strong
> Imbibes new life, and scours and stinks along.

(Pope had spasmodically a medical student sense of humour. In what other mood could he have written of George II's Queen Caroline's deathbed:

> Here lies wrapt up in forty thousand towels
> The only proof that Caroline had bowels.)

The eighteenth century produced also delightful pictures of kneeling bare-buttocked ladies attended by their

26. *The founder of the NHS, Chancellor von Bismarck.*

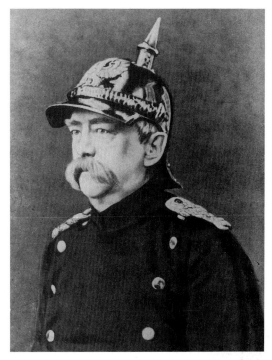

27. *Talking heads.*
The heads of Auguste and Abel Pollet, executed 1909.

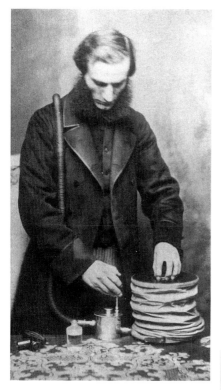

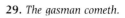
29. *The gasman cometh.*

28. *Dr Clover preparing
his chloroform.*

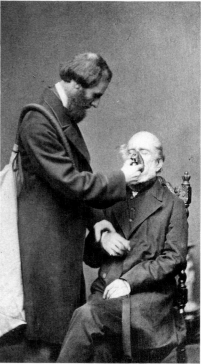

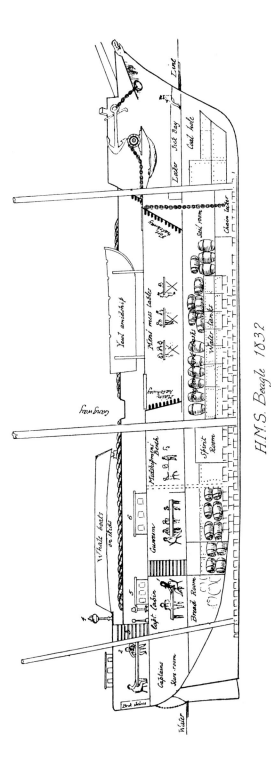

H.M.S. Beagle 1832

1 Mr Darwin's seat in Capt. Cabin
2   "   "   " Poop   "
3   "   "   drawers   "
4 Azimuth Compass
5 Captain's skylight
6 Gunroom   "

30. Darwin's Beagle.

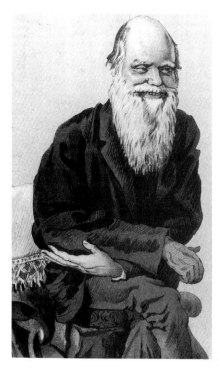

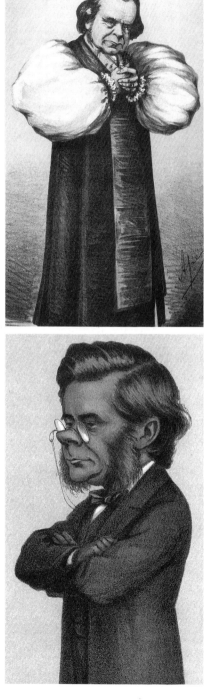

31. *Charles Darwin.*

32. *'Soapy Sam' Wilberforce.*

33. *Thomas Huxley.*

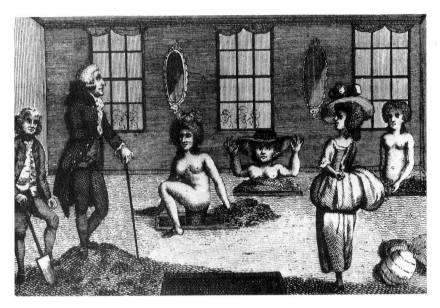

34. *Piccadilly earth baths.*

35. *Lady having enema.*

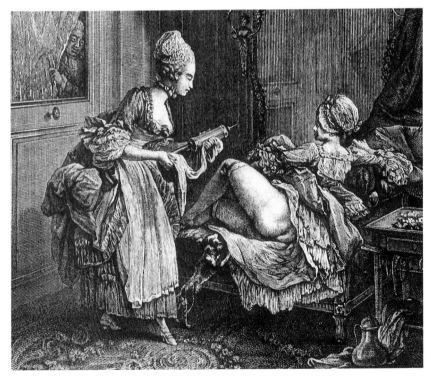

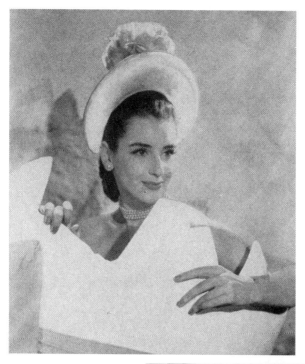

36. *Lovely Kay Kendall . . .*

37. *. . . lovelier after McIndoe nose job.*

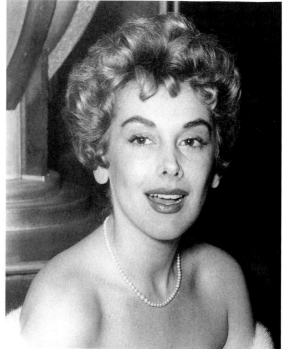

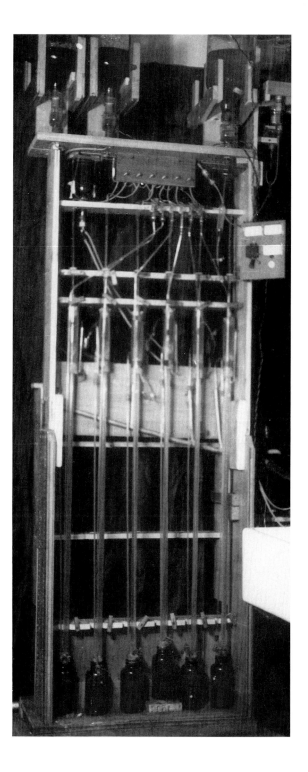

38. *The world's first penicillin factory.*

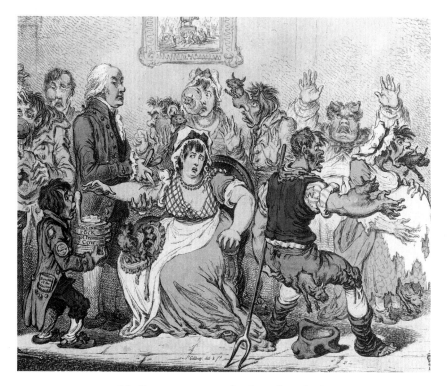

39. *Contemporary complications of vaccination.*

maids with seemingly nineteenth-century domestic fruit-sprays.

At the beginning of the twentieth century a conspiracy between patients and doctors engendered 'auto-intoxication'. Unspecified poisons were suspected of being absorbed from a sluggish colon, causing equally vague symptoms like cold clammy hands, cold bluish ears, lassitude, female pelvic pain and, according to Willie, a nasty graveyard odour. Though he added more cheerfully: 'In some peculiar manner red-haired people appear to possess a comparative immunity to the effects of intestinal stasis.' Lucky old Sarah Bernhardt.

A loaded colon incited Willie like a crammed butcher's window a starving revolutionary. It sometimes embodied 'Lane's kinks', which he steamed to iron out. His abdominal incision became ribs-to-pubis, right down the middle, to allow a better look at everything going on. He recommended oiling the colon with a daily pint of cream, and sleeping flat on the belly, emulating the African savages whose colons fired like General Kitchener's pompoms.

Willie was handsome, luxuriantly moustached, sarcastic, a leg-pulling Ulsterman, a keen ballroom dancer, a designer of his own instruments (which he liked hefty). He instructed:

> The English corset is disastrous in that it exerts a constricting encircling pressure on the abdomen about the lower costal margin and exaggerates the tendency to downward displacement of the viscera. The straight-busked French corset is much less harmful, and, if skilfully made and applied, serves to exert a moderate pressure on the lower abdomen.

You can tell that by comparing Renoir's women to Gainsborough's.

Then Willie met Ilya Mechnikoff (1845–1916) from Odessa. Professor Mechnikoff won the Nobel prize in 1908, and in 1903 wrote *La Vie Humaine*, a Balzacian title for his treatise proving the colon as unnecessary to the human body as wings for pigs. Revolutionary Willie instantly instituted a Reign of Terror, guillotining the colon at both ends and hurling it into the flames of the Guy's incinerator.

The colon was proscribed as a poisonous cess-pit, infecting the rest of the body with rheumatism, tuberculosis, cancer and lots of other things. A boy who mistook Willie's door for the throat clinic had his colon removed instead of his tonsils. A man who unsuccessfully cut his throat had not *his* colon removed but his wife's, to make her better-tempered and his home life happier.

The patients loved it, like Jove. It is comforting to identify inside you a whipping boy for all your physical and psychological imperfections.

A year later, the patients were back with the same symptoms which Willie had told them they had.

All this went on until 1913, when doctors began to suspect that the colon was loaded with nonsense. Spoke up Sir James Frederick Goodheart Bt (1845–1916), a Guy's physician:

> Encouraged by us doctors, hundreds of thousands of
> human beings have grafted into themselves the idea
> that they were born into the world for the main
> purpose of getting a daily evacuation of their bowels.

Willie retreated into olive oil, cod liver oil and liquid paraffin, of which 'I may safely assert that no remedy has rendered so much good to the human race.' He advised that we should abandon chairs, squatting with thighs pressed against belly, like those colonically-efficient savages. He directed his colleagues at Guy's to open their bowels twice a day. He founded the New Health Society, which involved writing for the newspapers, so in 1933 he struck himself off the medical *Register*. An obsessed man like Willie with the best intentions can do comparable harm to one like Bluebeard with the worst.

Willie was run over in the wartime blackout outside the Athenæum Club in Pall Mall, and died aged eighty-six still believing that the colon should forever be as empty as Mother Hubbard's cupboard. He had been extracting from it £10,000 a year. An old house-surgeon said Willie's work: 'Has a flavour of Celtic mysticism which perhaps betrays his Irish ancestry.' Perhaps it was all Willie's leg-pull.

Surgery à la mode

Patients who escaped from Willie with their colons risked equally ruthless treatment from equally energetic surgeons for their floating kidneys. These caused the same symptoms, by bobbing about the abdomen like balloons on New Year's Eve. Another intra-abdominal epidemic was of mysterious adhesions between the slippery organs, widely diagnosed and attacked with similar ferocity. They were later found to be fairly uncommon and mostly harmless, and anyway caused by the silicon talc powdering the surgeons' gloves. 'Ts & As' – tonsils and adenoids – was until the 1960s performed for such a miscellany of childhood ills that it became a routine ceremonial expurgation. Willie was surprisingly against this bloody, snatchy, dangerous operation, recommending instead breathing exercises, which his whole family did on their backs after tea.

The fashionable pathology of the 1920s was septic foci, pockets of pus lurking everywhere from the sinuses to the pelvis, expiated by busily slicing flesh and chipping bone. This delusion persisted until chemotherapy became the latest thing, and sepsis dropped out of fashion. After that, the vogue was operations for removing chains of sympathetic nerves, to abolish spasm of gut or arteries. Surgery without its cults would be as diminished as Paris without its collections.

Useless operations are being performed as widely and enthusiastically today, but unhappily nobody will know which ones they are until they have been abandoned for something else.

In a Flask Darkly

Seventeenth century painters were fond of depicting the solacers of Dutch interiors. Jan Steen of Delf's 'Physician's Visit' displays the pale daughter in her comfortable bedchamber, fortified by her anxious mother, while the smart doctor holds against the light a flask of her urine like an oenophile assessing the palatability of claret. David Teniers the Younger's 'Water Doctor' more fiercely inspects a flask just filled by a gloomy old woman with her shopping, and Gerard Dou's 'Mal d'Amour' has a pretty richly-dressed maiden and a handsome young befurred doctor, who is holding the pulse of her drooping wrist while both gaze at her urine with significant tenderness.

Uroscopy was the fashionable investigation, particularly for chlorosis. This was the green sickness, *morbo virgineo*, the bane of love-sick female puberty. Chlorosis was first described in 1554 by Johannes Lange (1485–1565), physician to the Elector of the Palatinate, when a friend's daughter was compelled thereby to refuse desirable suitors:

> Her face, which in the past year was distinguished by rosiness of cheeks and redness of lips, is somehow as if

exsanguinated, sadly paled, the heart trembles with every movement of her body, and the arteries of her temples pulsate, and she is seized with dyspnoea in dancing and climbing the stairs, her stomach loathes food and particularly meat, and the legs, especially at the ankles, become oedematous at night.

An admirable account of iron deficiency anaemia caused by the onset of menstruation and a faulty diet. His treatment: 'I instruct virgins afflicted with this disease, that as soon as possible they live with men and copulate.'

To uroscopists, the bulbous flask was the crystal ball, in which they could read anything. Inspecting urines pale, dark or frothy must nevertheless have instructed the shrewder ones about the equanimity of the kidney which produced them. London cardiologist Sir Thomas Lauder Brunton (1844–1916) recounted in 1892:

In the town of Leeds there once lived a quack who had received no professional instruction whatever, but was known far and wide for his wonderful cures, and especially for his power of diagnosing the diseases of patients whom he had never seen by simply examining their urine. A celebrated surgeon, Mr X, wishing to see his method of working, desired to be present one day, and the quack readily acceded to his request, feeling much flattered that so great a man should patronise him. Shortly after Mr X had taken his seat a woman came in with a bottle of urine, which she handed to the quack. He looked at her, then at the bottle, held it up between him and the light, shook it, and said, 'Your husband's?' 'Yes, sir.' 'He is a good deal older than you?' 'Yes, sir.' 'He is a tailor?' 'Yes, sir.' 'Here,' he said, handing her a box of pills, 'tell him to take one of these pills every night for a week and a big drink of cold water every morning and he will soon be all right.' No sooner had the woman gone out than Mr X turned to the quack, curious to know how he had made out all this. 'Well, you see,' said the quack, 'she was a young woman, and looked well and strong, and I guessed the water was not hers. I saw she had a wedding ring on her finger so I knew she was married, and I thought the chances were it was her husband's water. If he had been about the same age as she it was hardly likely that he was going to be ill either, so I guessed he was older. I knew he was a tailor because the bottle was stopped not with a cork, but with a bit of paper rolled up and tied round with thread in a way no one but a tailor could have done it. Tailors get no exercise, and consequently they are all very apt to be constipated. I was quite sure that he would be no exception to the rule and so I gave him opening pills.' 'But how did you know that she came from S.?' 'Oh, Mr X, have you lived so long in Leeds and don't know the colour of S. clay? It was the first thing I saw on her boots the moment she came in.'

Similarly, an Edinburgh surgeon in 1880 diagnosed a patient as a recently discharged sergeant from a regiment posted to Barbados: the man was respectful but forgetfully kept his hat on, as in the Army, he was Scottish with an air of authority, and he had elephantiasis, which you get in Barbados but not in the Highlands. Elementary, my dear Joseph Bell (1837–1911). As Arthur Conan Doyle (1859–1930) sat there as one of his students, Bell became Sherlock Holmes.

Uroscopists persisted to the middle of the nineteenth century, when the mysticism of urine evaporated from a newly perceived but unromantic solution of abundant and complex chemicals.

Bloody History

He told, that to these waters he had come
To gather leeches, being old and poor:
Employment hazardous and wearysome!

And he had many hardships to endure:
From pond to pond he roamed, from moor to moor;
Housing, with God's good help, by choice or chance;
And in this way he gained an honest maintenance,

wrote Wordsworth in 1807 of 'The Leech-gatherer', who had sable orbs of his yet-vivid eyes, he stirred the muddy waters about his feet, once he could meet with them on every side, but unhappily the leeches had gone off recently.

The leech was busily sucking away the ills of mankind from AD 900 until 1953, when they were applied to Stalin, but he died. Leeches may have been named after doctors, or doctors called after leeches, and 'to leech' meant to cure. St Luke's dig: 'Physician, heal thyself', is 'Leech leech yourself' in the Lindisfarne Gospels of AD 950, and in 1386 Chaucer was asking sensibly why anyone that had a 'parfit leche' need search for other leeches in the town.

The sanguivorous leech *Hirudo medicinalis* has a small head and a flat back or olive-green body with six yellow lines down it, and an ash-coloured speckled belly. It is one-and-a-half inches long, but expands to six on feeding. It has attachment suckers at both ends, ten stomachs down each side, an organ of taste (for blood) in the upper gullet, and a horseshoe-shaped mouth armed with three cartilaginous teeth, each said to stab like the triangular Italian dagger *estocado*. The leech has a female sexual orifice, also a penis in a sheath, but it hangs out when it is dead. *Hirudo medicinalis* is one of the world's 650 sorts of leech (the most powerful suckers are from the Amazon rain forests), and one of sixteen British ones, and is an officially endangered species.

In the history of blood-letting, leeches were taken from their water an hour before use to work up an appetite, placed in a wine glass and briskly upturned on to the flesh. After fifteen minutes they were gorged and dropped off, though they might go to sleep, but you could wake them up by splashing with cold water. To make them disgorge for recycling, sprinkle with salt. If short of leeches, the leecher snipped the tails off, and they would suck away with the blood flowing out of the other end, assumedly until the patient was exsanguinated. If they become stuck like a leech, their master wafted over them the fumes of burnt hair, or inserted a horsehair between sucker and host. If patient or physician inadvertently swallowed one, the antidote was shoemaker's blacking in vinegar.

Leeches were the cottage barometer, frisking in their open jar before rain and trying to flee from it before thunder. Medicinal leeches were eaten by horse leeches. In 1822 London imported from Bordeaux and Lisbon – with their more agreeable products – 7,200,000 leeches at half-a-crown apiece. We were still importing 2,000 a year at sixpence each in 1940. Since then, there was little call for them.

In 1825 France exported 10 million leeches and kept three million for home use. By 1833 France needed to import 41,500,000 leeches, through the exsanguinary energy of François-Joseph-Victor Broussais (1772–1838), a Breton who rose from sergeant to surgeon in Napoleon's Army. Like Willie Lane, he could diagnose only one disease: gastroenteritis. He particularised Scotsman John Brown's 'Brunonian System' (life depends on constant bodily stimulation), deciding that it was heat alone which unwontedly inflamed the body's chemicals. Broussais' cure was dousing the heat by fasting and applying leeches, fifty at a time, all over the skin. Broussais had shown an envied efficiency with the cutlass as a young soldier, and as a crusty old one urged on his followers to shed blood in torrents. They economised on leeches by slicing open the veins.

The leech was the physicians' pet because it was the mildest way of bleeding, suitable for women, children and paying patients. First-century Teuton warriors used their wives and mothers to suck their wounds even more gently. More vigorous blood-letting became the vogue of the seventeenth century, gore dripping into surgeons' pewter porringers, flattened on one side to nestle against the flesh, or into Venetian bleeding-glasses which were treasured as heirlooms. A man paid half-a-crown to be bled, but a lady in bed cost ten shillings. Poor King Charles II was an unconscionable and uncomfortable time dying, being bled, clystered, blistered, sweated and sicked. Bleeding, purging, puking and perspiring was the standard medical treatment, which diminished only with the diminishing years of the nineteenth century. Physicians had no idea what made their patients ill, but whatever it was, it seemed sensible somehow to get rid of it.

John Coakley Lettsom (1744–1815) was a Georgian physician so busy that he wore out three pair of horses a day, attending the 82,000 patients a year who brought him a £12,000 income, a house by the Guildhall and an estate in Kent. He was the son of a West Indian cotton-planter, who inherited interesting genetics: he was one of the only pair to survive from seven sets of twins.

Lettsom nobly liberated his material inheritance – Negro slaves – and went to Edinburgh to learn medicine. He enthusiastically founded the present London Medical Society in 1773, and a dozen benevolent institutions, including the Society for the Discharge and Relief of Persons Imprisoned for Small Debts, and – presciently – the Royal Humane Society for resuscitation of the apparently dead. He intelligently stood up for Jenner over vaccination. He was tall and gaunt, a drably-dressed

Quaker fond of wine and girls, who decently gave 'necessitous clergymen and literary men' free consultations. He ran his practice on the principles:

> When patients comes to I,
> I physics, bleeds, and sweats 'em;
> Then – if they choose to die,
> What's that to I? I Lettsom.

The leech has recently been revived for eating up the clots of plastic surgery and for scavenging bruises and black eyes.

Sad Ends

'Treatment', begins a medical textbook of 1904, reaching that section in the chapter on acute lobar pneumonia:

> The patient of necessity takes to his bed . . . the diet should consist of milk and beef-tea, or mutton broth administered in small quantities, frequently . . . in early stages the bowels should be opened . . .

It rambles on hopefully about:

> A few leeches or ice-applications, linseed-meal poultices which may be sprinkled with mustard, or hot flannels wrung out of turpentine . . . stimulants are probably our most important aids under the circumstances and brandy may be given to the extent of 4, 6, or 8 ounces daily.

It ends bleakly:

> The only hope of cutting short the disease lies in the discovery of an efficient anti-pneumococcus serum.

Until the late 1930s, medical textbooks instructing on pneumonia fussed away exactly like those of the 1900s. Even in the year of Pearl Harbor, an immaculately blue-dressed, crisp-aproned, frilly-hatted ward sister demonstrated to my student class 'dry cupping'. As elegantly as sewing samplers, she raised egg-sized mounds of patients' skin in wine-glasses vacuumised by heat, this being her favoured treatment of lung congestion, for which our current textbook still recommended the seventeenth century practice of bleeding and 'the application of 6 leeches over the liver'.

An anti-pneumococcus serum had been discovered, but the hopes of 1904 were misplaced. Sir Almroth Wright was summoned in 1911 to quell the constant pneumonia among the native workers of the Rand gold-mines – it was so wasteful for their white employers – and unsuccessfully tried to mirror in pneumonia the resplendent inoculation he had kindled against typhoid. As Sir Almroth was unable to *prevent* pneumonia, he armed himself in St Mary's Hospital between the wars with a serum, created from pneumonia-infected horses, to cure it instead.

But there were too many varieties of the pneumococcus germ for him to take accurate aim, and the weapon usually misfired anyway. Pneumonia remained 'the old man's friend', which swiftly and pityingly released him from the aches and miseries of age; but as abruptly it savagely killed his eighteen-year-old grandson, who was wrapped in a woolly pneumonia-jacket, isolated by a disinfected sheet hung across the door, straw spread outside to deaden the passing noise, and nothing much else which anyone could do for him. He gasped blue-faced towards the seventh day crisis, when the temperature fell and hope rose, or not. Pneumonia in the young was a cruel drama, because the tragedy was not inevitable.

In pneumonia the lung becomes solid, in tuberculosis –
phthisis, Greek for wasting – it develops holes. It generally announces itself with spat blood. 'I know the colour
of that blood! It is arterial blood. I cannot be deceived in
that colour. That drop of blood is my death warrant. I
must die,' John Keats (1795–1821) cried poignantly when
he suffered a haemoptysis.

Keats knew what he was talking about, having qualified at Guy's Hospital in 1816. His brother Tom died of
pulmonary tuberculosis in 1818, he had nursed his
mother before she died of it in 1810, he had the familial
susceptibility and the exposure. Anne, Emily and Charlotte Brontë coughed over each other in Yorkshire and
perished of it, so did Robert Louis Stevenson in Samoa,
D. H. Lawrence in Provence and George Orwell immediately he had finished *1984*. Dr William Somerset
Maugham (1874–1965), who qualified at St Thomas's in
1897, developed tuberculosis during World War One, but
– somehow, predictably – made both a full recovery and
wrote *Sanatorium*.

Sanatoriums in 1929 won the Nobel Prize – for Literature. Thomas Mann's *The Magic Mountain* detaches
characters who might be travelling first class on a trans-
atlantic liner but are travelling to eternity in the Swiss
Alps, their doctor the bright-and-breezy Hofrat striding
the bridge.

A sanatorium was a handy device for novelists, particularly as the occupants of the same sinking boat were
buoyed with *spes phthisica*, the mysterious symptomatic
hope, which springs eternal in a human breast which is
coughing copious sputum into capped pots like German
beer-mugs. Emotions stirred restlessly in the sanatorium's prescribed immobility, which was to be endured
both day and night in the open air. Everyone lay well

tucked-up on long steamer chairs, only careful meals and temperature-taking to pass the time with unremitting punctuality, release distant or improbable, and death an irritating gate-crasher to the cosy party.

The first tuberculosis sanatorium was opened by Hermann Brehmer (1826–99) in the Sudeten Mountains in 1859. Afterwards they sprang up regularly from Davos to the Adirondacks, most thickly in the spa-spangled Taunus Mountains rising from the Rhine. This hope of cold, fresh air healing the lungs was earlier expressed by the Royal Sea-bathing Hospital, which John Lettsom founded in 1796 for scrofulous children at Margate, a favourite resort of the hardy British holidaymaker.

The idea evolved that unbroken rest in chilly, rarefied air damped the fires of bodily metabolism and shallowed the breathing, so resting the inflamed lung and encouraging the cavities to close. The stay-at-home alternative was an artificial pneumothorax, filling the normally imperceptible space against the chest-wall with air through a needle, and collapsing the diseased lung.

Neither communal nor personal treatment of the lungs did much good. Nor did the fashionable, fanciful doses of cod-liver oil, creosote, iodine, arsenic and gold. The 'white plague' continued to reap: Chekhov, Chopin, Aubrey Beardsley, Katherine Mansfield, Modigliani, Kafka and Dr Laënnec who invented the stethoscope. It was 'The Consumption of Young Men, that are in the Flower of their Age, when the heat of the Blood is yet brisk,' as despondently seen by Richard Morton's (1637–98) *Phthisiologia* in 1689.

Jean-Antoine Villemin (1827–92), Professor at the French Army medical school at Val-de-Grâce, is credited with discovering in 1868 that tuberculosis was infective. He gave it to rabbits. But clear-sighted Dr Tobias Smollett, who was sensitive about infection, was persisting in 1771:

You won't deny, that many diseases are infectious; even the consumption itself is highly infectious. When a person dies of it in Italy, the bed and bedding are destroyed; the other furniture is exposed to the weather, and the apartment white-washed, before it is occupied by any other living soul. You'll allow, that nothing receives infection sooner, or retains it longer, than blankets, feather-beds, and mattresses. 'Sdeath! how do I know what miserable objects have been stewing in the bed where I now lie!

Professor Villemin himself indicated usefully: 'The phthisical soldier is to his messmate what the glandered horse is to its yokefellow.' But that was fourteen years before Koch identified the tubercule bacillus, and before Pasteur had got into his stride, so nobody took any notice.

Happy End

Pneumonia's ageless therapies have vanished, like the quaint hospital superstitions of mixing red and white flowers (they foretell a death), or leaving flowers in the wards overnight (they consume the oxygen), or hanging the 'danger list' upon the hospital entrance ('On the gate and dying nicely,' an Irish ward sister would enlighten the houseman of a patient's condition).

Many treatments of desperate futility disappeared during the 1940s, like the paraphernalia of coaching before steam, the agony of operations before anaesthetics, or the regular slaughter of world wars before their outlawry by the mutual terror of the H-bomb. You could now have pneumonia in your own home. The Swiss could turn their sanatoriums into hotels, to be complimented on their deep balconies with extensive views, available in all rooms for after-lunch snoozing in the crisp sunshine.

Septicaemia, diphtheria, typhoid, typhus, gonorrhea, erysipelas and other deadly serpents in our Garden of Eden were snared with antibiotics. Man's ingenuity even adapted his drugs to outmatch the new resistance of their resourceful foes. Effective medicine began on Christmas Eve 1932, when Domagk in the Rhineland saw that those mice infected with streptococci, but dosed with sulphanilamide, would live to see Christmas Day.

End of an Argument?

Without animal experiments like Domagk's, conducted under law and with the humanity that, lacking, would leave us without any doctors at all, these drugs would not have achieved our wonderment. Anti-vivisectionists, more muddled in their heads than cruel towards their suffering fellow-humans, need not agree with Aldous Huxley:

> I'm not one of those fools who think that one life is as good as another, simply because it *is* a life; that a grasshopper is as good as a dog and a dog is as good as a man. You must recognize a hierarchy of existences.

But they do need to note a defence put forward for Professor Heinrich Hörlein, Domagk's boss, on trial at Nürnberg in 1948:

> He took part in the fight for freedom in the field of science, against the plans of Hitler and Göring to prohibit vivisection for scientific purposes.

You can tell an idealist by the company he keeps.

NINE

Odd Practices

Medicine, like politics, is a powerful magnet for weighty convictions of false metal.

Home Medicine

Cures once rumoured as infallible:

- 1. *Paediatric hernias.* Strip the child, find a young pollard-ash, split it longitudinally and hold it open by wedges, push child through, plaster tree with loam and swathe tightly. But if the cleft continues to gape, so does the hernia. Practised in Selborne in 1776, though Gilbert White uncharitably cut down the swathed trees to enlarge his garden.
- 2. *Warts.* Touch each wart with a separate pebble, put pebbles in bag, drop bag on way to church, finder will

start sprouting your warts. Or seek a man who never saw his father and ask to touch his coat. As prophylaxis, never let your children touch the water of boiled eggs.

— 3. *Mumps*. Take the halter from the ass, noose the patient and lead him round the pig-sty. Repeat three times.

— 4. *Whooping cough*. Drink water from the skull of a bishop, if available. One was, in 1830 in Co Cavan. In Co Cork, sheep droppings boiled in milk was a valued draught. Or catch a fish, hold its head in the patient's mouth, and you can then return it to the river with the disease. Or pass the patient under and over a donkey, repeating nine times.

— 5. *Potato therapy*. For a cold, hang a stocking filled with hot potatoes round the neck, or rub a roast one in the head. A raw potato in the pocket prevents rheumatism. If it fails, sleep with the dog, who will absorb the rheumatism and become crippled, though the RSPCA may become annoyed. For sexual stamina, crush raw potato, carrots, cabbage and mint (it did wonders for the Queen of Sheba; and it clarified to an American herbalist the English propensity for spooning mint sauce on the lamb and potatoes). Potatoes with garden peas are contraceptive (well, they reduce the fertility of rats), though Mexican women prefer yams. A potato rub-down is an easier way of shedding warts.

— 6. *Charming ways*. Sir Walter Scott's Talisman was the amulet by which the Saladin, disguised as a physician, cured the crusading Richard I. It ended up as a red stone in an Edward IV coin possessed by the Lockharts of the Lee in Lanarkshire, the 'Lee Penny', so powerful that its mere dipping-in rendered any water highly curative. When Newcastle town borrowed it for an epidemic under Charles I, they had to put up £6,000 as security. Preventative measures against disease demanded the acquisition of coffin nails, snake skins, a hare's right front paw, and — particularly against poisoning — the bezoar stone, a concretion from the guts of the wild goat of Persia (from the Peruvian llama, less effective). Red was the curative colour, red flannel for sore throats, a decent Burgundy for anaemia. The 'powder of sympathy' was but copper sulphate, applied curatively in the mid-seventeenth century to the weapon, not the wound. Intelligent people still wear copper bracelets to ward off rheumatism and such ills, as hopefully and futilely as enjoying unrequited love.

Taking the Waters

What would eighteenth-century English literature have done without Bath? 'Oh! who can ever be tired of Bath?' gushed Jane Austen, efficiently using it as a location for *Northanger Abbey*. Bath was a delightful backdrop, readily inviting a powerful plot congregating a large cast of intelligent, witty, crotchety, worldly, amorous characters. Fielding, Fanny Burney, Sheridan, Oliver Goldsmith, Robert Southey, Walter Savage Landor, William Cowper, Wordsworth and Walter Scott all dipped into Bath. Why, Bath bubbled along like a modern soap!

In 1830, Mr Pickwick took upstairs rooms for two months in Royal Crescent, to forget Bardell *v* Pickwick. He drank a quarter-pint of the waters before and after breakfast, and solemnly declared that he felt a great deal better: 'Whereat his friends were very much delighted, though they had not been previously aware that there was anything the matter with him'.

Sam Weller's famous opinion of the waters: 'They'd a wery strong flavour o' warm flat irons'.

Bath's daily half-million gallons spout at 120°F. Visitors can easefully splash in it, or conscientiously swallow it, but neither produces any beneficial medical effect. Like the waters springing from other delightful corners of Europe, their dissolved minerals are an unnecessary addition to the normal dietetic intake, and their warm caress affords but a flirtatious soothing.

Tobias George Smollett (1721–1771) had been a practitioner in Bath, where his lack of success was succeeded by his lack of popularity in writing *An Essay on the External Use of Water*, implying that the waters of Bath were no more miraculous than water anywhere else. He analysed them in *Humphry Clinker* in 1771:

> The water contains nothing but a little salt, and calcarious earth, mixed in such inconsiderable proportion, as can have very little, if any, effect on the animal oeconomy. This being the case, I think the man deserves to be fitted with a cap and bells, who, for such a paltry advantage as this spring affords, sacrifices his precious time, which might be employed in taking more effectual remedies.

He added that bathing in it was to risk 'the king's evil, the scurvy, the cancer, and the pox'. He did not care for Bath's architecture, either.

'Smelfungus' Smollett was right. But so was Mr Pickwick. It is always agreeable to feel better, even if you are not.

The Romans built Bath, but its Baron Haussmann was gamester Richard 'Beau' Nash, who, according to Oliver Goldsmith, habitually travelled in a post-chariot drawn by six greys, with outriders, footmen and French horns, and who founded the Assembly Rooms and inspired John Wood to design the lovely limestone squares, streets and crescents. Nash was a difficult patient:

> The next day, when the physician called and enquired if his prescription had been followed, the beau languidly replied, 'No, i'faith, doctor, I haven't followed it. 'Pon honour, if I had I should have broken my neck, for I threw it out of my bedroom window.'

As the King of Bath, Nash led the extravagant balls, insisted that everyone behaved and dressed decently, supervised the young ladies' morals and got rid of the footpads, and like Baron Haussmann in Paris he died in 1762 impoverished. His joke survived him, to become a caricature caption on 20 December 1797.

An Act of Parliament in 1597 had bestowed the 'right to the free use of the baths of Bath to the diseased and impotent poor of England,' but these inconvenient Beggars of Bath were tidied away by its repeal in 1714. In the eighteenth century, the Pump Room offered fashionable drinkers the fashionable cure for rheumatism and gout, and for anything else that struck their sickly fancy. In the murky dawn of scientific medicine the next century, the reputation of curative natural waters slowly dissolved. Though people continued to travel significant distances on the novel railways to take the waters at spas, because it is agreeable to partake of painless treatment amid pleasant surroundings, in the company of fellow-sufferers to whom it is socially acceptable to impart your symptoms at length.

The Greeks had the spa idea in 8 BC with the cult of 'incubation', which is sleeping in Asklepieia, the temples of the God of Healing. The patients journeyed to Cos or Pergamos or Athens, sacrificed a ram, had a bath, and slept in sympathetic togetherness among the pillars open to the darkness. During the night, Aesculapius materialised in dazzling light, snakes licked your eyelids, and in the morning you went home cured. Resistant patients stayed on, drinking and bathing in the springs, taking the diet, massage and exercise. The cost was presenting a replica of your diseased part, in silver or gold. Aesculapius was really the local priest, stage-managing the visions and performing a repertoire of minor cures. The system has been preserved precisely at Lourdes, which cures nobody but provides a businesslike organisation to slake human hope and douse despair with the water of sparkling illusion.

The subterranean torrents of the spas flowed on, to irrigate today's equally untherapeutic health farms. A similar *camaraderie*, reinforced by everyone paying the atrocious fees, sustains a regimen of rigorous abstinence that admirably and pridefully reduces body weight, an effect which persists a month or two after release into the delightful social obligations to gluttony. The diets which nourish health farms and flesh out magazines and newspapers are superfluous. The secret of losing weight is simple and costless: eat less and booze nothing.

One enduring good came from the eighteenth century Bath medical establishment. Dr William Oliver (1695–1764) left to his trusty coachman Atkins the recipe for the crisp, thin, pitted, white, dry biscuit which he had created. With support from Beau Nash, Oliver had founded the Bath Mineral Water Hospital in 1742, and wrote *A Practical Essay on the Use and Abuse of Warm Bathing in Gouty Cases*. He died from gout. A snappy Bath Oliver will do you all the good of the Bath waters, particularly with a mound of ripe stilton, a jar of crisp celery, some pickled walnuts and a glass of port.

Taking the Mud

Handsome, androgenic James Graham (1745–94), former Edinburgh medical student, was among the fattest quacks to peck at the hardy shoots of human credulity over the centuries. (A quack is the mid-seventeenth century abbreviation of 'quacksalver', a man who boasts about his salves.) About 1780, Graham opened his earth-baths in London off the Haymarket. An engraving depicts four naked ladies in modish hats climbing into square pits under his masterful eye, with a boy to shovel in the soil. Such fangotherapy returned in the 1930s as the facial mud-pack, which sadly does nothing for the face. A curiosity of Isherwood's Berlin to survive the Nazis and the War was women wrestling in mud. They wore swimsuits and rubber bathing-hats, spectators in the front stalls were issued with long splashproof bibs, and some time in the contest a tit or two had to pop out.

Graham ran London's first infertility clinic, utilising the Celestial Bed at his Temple of Health, which stood in the newly built Adelphi beside the Thames. The Bed was the size of a snooker-table, 'in brocaded damask supported by four crystal pillars of spiral shape festooned with garlands of flowers in gilded metal'. It was perfumed with Arabian spices, and in the next room the orchestra kept on playing. The silk sheets were purple and the mattress stuffed with hair from the tails of English stallions.

You could tilt the bed to taste, while streams of light played over a canopy presenting the figures of Cupid, Psyche and Hymen, and a pair of live turtle doves. The operative bit was fifteen hundredweight of magnets underneath. It cost £100 a go. 'The superior ecstasy which the parties enjoy in the Celestial bed is really astonishing and never before thought of in this world,' Graham guaranteed. 'The barren certainly must become fruitful when they are powerfully agitated in the delight of love.' In the morning, he took the couple's pulses and gave them breakfast, then 'sends them away full of hope, not forgetting to recommend them to send him other clients.'

The Temple of Health (admission six guineas), which soon moved to fashionable Pall Mall, was all mirrors, dazzling lights, flaming dragons, hidden music and wafted perfumes. It offered magnetised baths 'to dissipate melancholy and mitigate extravagant gaiety'. It flourished its testimonials:

Over the doors of the principal rooms, under the vaulted compartments of the ceiling, and in each side of the centre arches of the hall, are placed walking-sticks, ear-trumpets, visual glasses, crutches, &c. left, and here placed as the most honourable trophies, by deaf, weak, paralytic, and emaciated persons, cripples, &c., who, being cured, have happily no longer need of such assistance.

A century later, the Grotto of Lourdes used the same plug. 'What! No wooden legs?' murmured Anatole France.

The robed Graham gave lectures, with the startling climax of electric shocks for the whole audience from wires hidden under the cushions. Electricity had then arrived in real medicine, the patients in London hospitals being shocked hopefully for almost everything. Graham was supported by diaphanously draped Goddesses of Health, one of whom, Emma Lyons, did well for herself as Nelson's Lady Hamilton.

James Graham had practised his sort of medicine in Philadelphia and in Bath. In 1779, at Aix-la-Chapelle, he had treated the Duchess of Devonshire, a notably soft touch for quacks, who enjoyed it so much that she projected him into London society. In 1782 London society tumbled him. The Temple was closed, the Bed sold to some eternally blissful couple, Graham returned to Edinburgh, was imprisoned in the Tollbooth for libelling the magistrates, got religion, went mad, and 'remained naked in the earth for several hours on nine successive days'. His mud failed him, and he died.

Graham should have stuck to his ancillary recommendations of open windows, fresh air, exercise, frugal diet and timorous drinking:

Port wine is certainly one of the greatest bracers or holders together of the incorporated cattle of Great

Britain! The great curdler and feast vomit of those too
numerous all-devouring herds! and which is,
moreover, one of the principal causes of gout, gravel,
rheumatism, asthmas, and apoplexies!

He would have enjoyed the reverence of a medical
John the Baptist, the forerunner by two centuries of the
austere teachings of the Royal College of Physicians.
But who would have listened to him?

A Soft Touch

1660 was a busy year for Charles II. He touched 6,725 of
his newly-restored subjects for the King's Evil. This was
scrofula, tuberculous infection of the chain of lymph
glands in the neck, which creates swellings between the
angle of the jaw and the top of the breastbone. Nothing
much could be done about it until the invention of
streptomycin, for which Professor Shelman Abraham
Waksman (1888–1973) of Rutgers University won the
Nobel Prize in 1952 (in 1941, he invented also the word
'antibiotics').

Charles II was as enthusiastic for the Royal Touch as
for the royal mistresses. His reign bestowed it on 92,107
kneeling patients, from a canopied throne flanked by
clergy and courtiers with a double file of halberded
Beefeaters as receptionists. Victorian medical historian
John Cordy Jeafferson (1831–91) pondered about:

> The inspiriting sensations experienced by a troop of
> wretches taken from their kennels to Whitehall, and
> brought into personal contact with the sovereign –
> their idea of grandeur!

While reminding his readers of Montaigne:

These apes' tricks are the main cause of the effect, our fancy being so far seduced as to believe that such strange and uncouth formalities must of necessity proceed from some abstruse science. Their very inanity gives them reverence and weight.

Everyone departed clutching the 'touchpiece' of a specially minted gold angel, which brought them more realistic benefit.

Edward the Confessor had initiated the touching treatment about 1045, though Clovis in AD 494 established it in France with a popularity that lasted until Charles X touched 121 patients at his coronation in 1824 – the year that science, through Sadi Carnot, had established the second law of thermodynamics. The cure died in England with Queen Anne, who touched Samuel Johnson, aged two, without success. William III had touched a few, but with the admirable invocation: 'God grant you better health and more sense.'

The mechanism of this remedy was God acting through divine right. Chubby Irishman Valentine Greatrakes (1628–66), an old Cromwellian soldier, saw no reason why God should not act through himself. He transmitted the healing effluvia arising from the ferments of his body by gentle stroking, though he used carrot poultices as well. Franz Anton Mesmer (1734–1815) from Switzerland revived the therapy, after discovering that he was charged with animal magnetism.

Mesmerising

Mesmer was a respectable physician in Vienna enjoying a rich wife and musical evenings with the Mozarts, until he met Professor Maximilian Hell, who knew how to cure people with magnets. Mesmer swiftly discarded the magnets, finding he could magnetise everything with his fingertips: men, women, dogs, his *Apfeltasche*. 'I myself magnetised the sun some twenty years ago,' he explained modestly to a doctor inquiring why he had ordered open-air bathing.

In 1778, one of Maria Theresa's commissions investigated Mesmer's practice and gave him twenty-four hours to leave Vienna. It was a boostful emigration. After dallying at Spa he moved to Paris, where in rue Montmartre he hypnotised ladies while wearing a lilac suit, playing the harmonica and waving a wand. His clinic in the Hotel Bullion, like James Graham's in Pall Mall, was furnished with carpets, mirrors, hidden music and wafted incense. It had magnetic tubs which the ladies pressed against, holding hands, until the entry of the assistant magnetisers. These were strong, handsome young men who 'embraced the patients between the knees', and rubbed them along the spine, down the neck, and on their breasts. It occasioned sobbing, tearing of the hair, laughter, shrieking, screaming, fits and insensibility. Serious cases saw Mesmer in his room, alone.

He had his failures. The only hope for M Campan with pneumonia was one of three remedies which were laid beside him in bed: a young woman of brown complexion, a black hen, and an old bottle. 'Sir,' Mme Campan urged Mesmer, 'if the choice be a matter of indifference, pray try the empty bottle,' but it didn't work. Louis XVI appointed his own investigating commission, though Marie Antoinette thought Mesmer was lovely. 'L'imagination fait tout, le magnétisme nul,' the commission complimented him. Mesmer left with the Revolution.

The animal magnetism that powered Mesmer's hypnotism invigorated John Elliotson (1791–1868) in London, who threw the sisters young Elizabeth and Jane O'Key into a trance and drew them round the room after him with a magnet. He adopted phrenology, diagnosing character from the shape of the head, which is like assessing the performance of a second-hand car by feeling the bonnet. This did not go down well with the medical profession, as Elliotson at the time occupied the first Chair of Medicine at University ('Godless', ie not exclusively for C of E) College, from which he was unseated in 1838. He had an outlasting compensation:

A kind friend brought you to my bedside, whence, in all probability, I should never have risen but for your constant watchfulness and skill . . . and as you would take no other fee but thanks, let me record them here,'

wrote W. M. Thackeray in 1850, dedicating to him *Pendennis.*

Scotsman James Esdale (1808–59) of the Indian Medical Service, in 1845 successfully hypnotised 261 Hindu convicts for surgical operations, but returning home found the Scots less susceptible. The desperate hope of mesmerism to abate the agony of surgery was anyway joyously blown away the following year by the vapour of ether. Another Scotsman, James Braid (1795–1861), had suspected hypnotism of 'collusion and illusion'. He found that trance could envelop any impressionable subject staring at anything bright. Illustrious neurologist Jean-Martin Charcot (1825–93) at the Salpêtrière Hospital in Paris successfully hypnotised young women with hysterical paralytic symptoms, towards which he noticed they strangely displayed *la belle indifférence.* Charcot was a showman, the distinction between the patient and the actress, and between the physician and the producer, more supple than they should have been. His audience in 1886 contained young Freud, portentously. Hypnotism is still used for snuffing suggestible smokers.

Small, goateed Émile Coué (1857–1926) of Nancy extended hypnotism to the mass market by calling it auto-suggestion. He would enjoin a hallful of mostly female votaries to clasp their hands and exclaim: 'Every day and in every way I am getting better and better.' He added that if they wanted to unclasp their hands they could not, and he was right. 'Think now: "I can",' he directed, and they could. This rewarded him with a worldwide reputation, until in London in 1922 the audience turned hysterical and he had to bolt. Hypnotism continued as a similar music hall act with malleable volunteers from the audience, until it was killed like the jugglers and performing seals by television.

Herbalism

Sick dogs eat grass. Sick man was able more intelligently to select herbs to alleviate his several pains, while shunning those liable to poison him. The optimistic abundance of these culled remedies invited classification by Pedacius Dioscorides (AD 54–68), a Greek surgeon marching with Nero's army. His *De Materia Medica Libri Quinque* was so successful that it went on selling for sixteen centuries. The herbal was the physician's weaponry. By the reign of Elizabeth I, these books flowered into delicate coloured pictures of plants, which their authors grew in aromatic profusion.

The herbalist, astrologer and Cromwellian Nicholas Culpeper's wildly popular *English Physician* of 1653 prescribes over 500 plants, from agrimony to yucca, to clear a dense thicket of human ills from adder bites to wind. Culpeper was the bad fairy at the bottom of the herb garden. The Royal College of Physicians had published a Latin *Pharmacopæia* in 1618, its 2,140 remedies including dried viper lozenges, foxes' lungs, live frogs, wolf oil and crabs' eyes, later editions adding hanged man's skull, human urine and placenta, swallows' nests and Irish whiskey. In his own *Physical Directory* of 1649 Culpeper cribbed the *Pharmacopæia*, translated it into English, and mocked it. The College was outraged:

> By two yeeres drunken labour he hath Gallimawfred the apothecaries book into nonsense . . . and (to supply his drunkenness and leachery with a thirty shilling reward) endeavoured to bring into obloquy the famous societies of apothecaries and chyrurgeons.

The split between herbalism and medicine had opened. It widened steadily but less explosively until the General Medical Council published the first *British Pharmacopæia* in 1864, which is now the paperback *British National Formulary* in every houseman's white-coat pocket. The mystery has been extracted from herbalism by biochemists: it has been synthesised and standardised, as morphine from the poppy, digitalis from the foxglove, and anti-scurvy ascorbic acid from lemons. Herbs are but fossils buried below the rich mine of man-made drugs that we so gratefully and busily work.

Herbalists persist today, expressing their quaint belief that nature's plants are somehow better than man's concoctions. They quote herbal tonics that did wonders for old ladies, which is understandable as they were dissolved in alcohol with a strength approaching gin. They gleefully cite disasters like thalidomide to prove that chemical cures have horrible unknown dangers. Quite right. If flying had been abandoned after the first plane crash, the world's plight would be tolerable, compared to the abandonment of scientific remedies in favour of the flowers that bloom in the spring, tra-la.

The Nazis were fanatical herbalists, warmly encouraged by Julius Streicher, whom we hung in 1946.

'Damn your bloods, don't you know me? I am Mrs Mapp, the bonesetter!' shouted 'Crazy Sally' from her coach-and-four with the gorgeously liveried footmen in the Old Kent Road. She was 'dressed in a loosely-fitting robe-de-chambre, and manifesting by her manner that she had partaken somewhat too freely of Geneva water', and had been mistaken by a threatening mob for one of George II's resented mistresses. Such quick-witted identification, like Nell Gwyn's earlier 'I am the Protestant whore', upturned a crowd's anger to loud applause.

Everybody in London knew fat and ugly Sally Mapp. There was a song about her in the play at Lincoln's Inn Fields, *The Husband's Relief*. Her sister Lavinia was the rage of 1728 as Polly Peachum in *The Beggar's Opera*, then she did Ophelia and married the third Duke of Bolton. Sally performed consultations twice weekly at the Grecian Coffee House. In 1736, she was paid 100 guineas a year by Epsom to live there and set fashionable bones. She married a footman who beat her for a fortnight then decamped with her money, she died in obscurity and poverty at Seven Dials, and lives forever at the top of Hogarth's portrait of massed bewigged, gold-headed cane sniffing physicians, *The Undertakers*.

Sir Hans Sloane, then President of the College of Physicians, applauded her:

> The cures of the woman bonesetter of Epsom are too
> many to be enumerated: her bandages are
> extraordinary neat, and her dexterity in reducing
> dislocations and setting fractured bones wonderful, she
> has cured persons who have been twenty years
> disabled.

Percival Pott gave her a bleaker notice:

We all remember that even the absurdities and impracticability of her own promises and engagement were by no means equal to the expectations and credulity of those who ran after her; that is of all ranks and degrees of people from the lowest labourer or mechanic up to those of the most exalted rank and station; several of whom not only did not hesitate to believe implicitly the most extravagant assertions of an ignorant illiberal drunken female savage, but even solicited her company; at least seemed to enjoy her society.

These two opinions crystallise the medical profession's relationship with osteopathy, which was invented in 1874 by Dr Andrew Taylor Still (1828–1917) in Kansas City. He decided that all illness flowed from derangement of the bodily structure, which he had learnt on Red Indians 'resurrected' by mid-Western Burke and Hares. Manipulate the misalignments and the patients recover, he said. He came to the attention of our House of Lords in 1934, when Still's noble enthusiasts wanted a lawful register of osteopaths, as of doctors. The Select Committee, into which the Bill was shunted by top medical Lords Dawson and Moynihan, shared the doctors' horror at Parliament licensing osteopaths to diagnose and treat human disease. 'It would not be safe or proper,' the Committee decided snubbingly.

This poured cold realism on the fuss about Herbert Atkinson Barker (1869–1950), son of the Lancashire coroner, uneducated beyond school, who made a packet as a fashionable London bonesetter and got a knighthood from Lloyd George in 1922. Barker then had the wind of Lord Beaverbrook's *Daily Express* at his back, which fanned public excitement at his anaesthetist being struck off the *Register* in 1911 for assisting an unqualified practitioner, and the military's refusal for him to treat the wounded in 1917. The Archbishop of Canterbury, who enjoys this ancient power, was clamoured to create Barker MD Lambeth, though this divine intervention would not have solemnised Barker's legal marriage to the General Medical Council.

'He had the gift of healing,' accords the *Dictionary of National Biography* to Herbert Barker. Would that anyone had. It is no giveaway, but accrued by intelligence and hard work.

A Drop in the Ocean

Dr John Brown (1735–88) of Edinburgh, a former theologian, solved the mystery of life. Life occurred, and continued, from stimulation of the excitable human body by food, movement, heat, emotion, thought and suchlike. If the stimulation was unduly increased, it gave us 'sthenic' diseases, treatable by sedation. If it lessened, we got 'asthenic' ones, demanding excitement. This was the 'Brunonian System' which so divided European medical opinion that the Hanoverian horse were called out in 1802 to quell a two-day riot at the University of Göttingen. Brown's treatment was opium and alcohol, lots of it. He dosed himself with wine, five glasses in quick succession, but it disprovingly killed him. He was later ungratefully asserted to have killed more people than the French Revolution and the Napoleonic Wars combined.

The reaction to Brown was Samuel Christian Friedrich Hahnemann (1755–1843) of Leipzig, who in 1810 invented homeopathy. He decided that drugs should be taken only in doses that were hardly noticeable. Like Paracelsus, he was a hair-of-the-dog man: if belladonna gives you scarlet spots, you give belladonna for scarlet fever. More soundly, he declared that only one cure should be given at once.

The homeopathic doctrine travelled powerfully to

America, where it was later dissected by Dr Oliver Wendell Holmes as 'a mingled mass of perverse ingenuity, of tinsel erudition, of imbecile credulity and of artful misrepresentation'. Despite which, its fabricator died in Paris a millionaire. Hahnemann's adherents still exist in the medical profession like doubting clerics, their church the Royal London Homeopathic Hospital. If our Queen is a homeopathic believer, this is in the majestic tradition. When Queen Adelaide consulted a homeopath, William IV ordered royal physician Robert Keate (1777–1857):

> 'Will you overhaul the prescription of the medicine which he orders for her, to see if she can safely take it?'
> I promised to do so, and on the prescription being handed to me, I said: 'Oh, your Majesty, she may take it for seven years, and at the end of that time she will not have taken a grain of medicine.'

Royalty is as liable to quirks as anyone else: we all have the same body, as Henry V complains moodily the night before Agincourt.

Science Fiction

Alternative medicine demands to be seen in perspective. Whereat it disappears beneath the horizon.

'Alternative' is the fashionable word to make the meaningless sound meaningful. It embellishes a mixture of medieval mysticism, herbalist nonsense, dietetic garbage, electrical toys, superstition, suggestion, ignorance and plain fraud.

You can try aromatherapy which smells nice, dance therapy which is fun, yoga and meditation which make for a relaxed evening, iridology if there are convenient eyes worth gazing into, palmistry which submits your fate to the fibrous skin bands of your hand, exorcism if you can persuade the vicar, and Christian Science if you want to live dangerously.

You can conjure from the dragon-smoke of Chinese history the life-forces of yin and yang and stab them, effecting with acupuncture the counter-irritation of an old-fashioned mustard plaster, which doctors once slapped on every bust, belly and bum in the practice. You can send a drop of your blood – or of your cat's blood – to a 'black box' with dials and knobs which will return you a diagnosis. This instrument was upheld in the High Court in 1960 because its inventor believed in it, exemplifying the odd legal principle that if you think you are innocent you must be.

'Is it really safe for me to go to a practitioner without medical qualifications?' asks one richly illustrated guide to alternative health. And replies: 'It is tempting, here, to suggest that you ask yourself instead the question, "How safe is it to go to my doctor?" Today's drugs are so powerful that if anything goes wrong, you may find the effects of the remedy worse than the disease. On balance, natural medicine is safer simply because it places less reliance on drugs.'

Dear me.

If you are ill, you compel scientific treatment. The only illnesses which 'healers' heal are those that their imaginative customers do not possess.

Medicine's relation to quackery is of astronomy to astrology. What the stars foretell for newspaper readers is harmless, but a space shuttle or a satellite directed by astrology in preference to astronomy would make a disastrous launch. But humans suffer an ageless susceptibility for quacks. Perhaps because everyone likes to think he knows better than his doctor. Perhaps because:

The patient, like a drowning man, catches at every
twig and hopes for relief from the most ignorant when
the most able physicians give him none,

as the *Spectator* noticed on 26 July 1714.
Perhaps because:

It has this enormous advantage over science that the
love of mystery is deeply implanted in the human
breast,

as the *BMJ* suggested in 1911.
Perhaps because:

The world is generally averse
To all the truths it sees and hears;
But swallows nonsense and a lie
With greediness and gluttony,

as observed by Samuel Butler.
Perhaps because, as Pliny sighed:

Minus credunt quae ad suam salutem pertinent, si
intelligunt. (People have less belief in things relating
to their health if they understand.)

Foretold Dr Carl Reinhold August Wunderlich
(1815–77) of Leipzig in 1858:

If the physician should sometimes suffer from
injustice and misunderstanding, should his honest
work now and then be ignored or even sneered at, he
must bear in mind that in the majestic eye of Nature
the individual is nothing. And however depressed he
may feel when intriguers and mountebanks blow
about their ephemeral successes, he may be sure that
these upstarts will be overtaken, in the end, by the
Erinyes of conscience. For natural science is a proud,

silently advancing power, of whose might the spheres most threatened by it have hardly a notion.

Do not tarry with the beachcombers on the wilder shores of science.

TEN

Freud, the English Governess and the Smell of Burnt Pudding

Between 1905 and 1914 Sigmund Freud (1856–1939) published from Vienna four case histories to establish unto an ignorant, indifferent or slightingly shrugging medical world the seriousness of his original insight into human personality.

Dora, Little Hans, the Rat Man and the Wolf Man

Eighteen-year-old Dora wanted to commit suicide, to revenge herself on her family, and on life, both of which failed to understand her. Her father (whom Freud had treated unpsychiatrically for syphilis) coveted his neighbour's wife. His neighbour coveted Dora. Dora's mother was chilly and remote, and more interested in the *Küche* than the *Kinder*. So Dora identified herself with the neighbour's wife, and fell in love with her father. Straightforward Oedipus stuff!

After three months of invoking her vanished dreams and unravelling her homespun tangles under psychoanalysis, Dora transferred her incestuous love to Freud. Then she broke it off. She vanished, saying she felt better. But she was not really better, Freud reasoned consolingly. She was merely experiencing a 'flight into health'. Freud's analytic treatment was publicly attacked next spring as 'mental masturbation', which were strong words to hear in Baden-Baden. The uncompleted case left Freud shaking his head for years. Poor Dora later tried a rival psychiatrist, but died sexually frigid, unmarried and unloved, if from natural causes.

Five-year-old Little Hans kicked and screamed rather than go for his morning walk in the park, because he was afraid that the horses might bite him. This eminently reasonable refusal was a barricade for his secret motive, which was seized by Freud. The case offers classic dialogue from the immense Freudian *œuvres*:

> MOTHER: (*Undressing.*) What are you staring like that for?
> HANS: I was only looking to see if you'd got a widdler, too.
> MOTHER: Of course. Didn't you know that?
> HANS: No, I thought you were so big you'd have a widdler like a horse.

This notion needed but little elaboration for Freud to establish that Little Hans was frightened of his father, who had a bigger widdler than his, and that Little Hans wished to insert his widdler into mummy, so he transferred his fear to horses, who had terrific widdlers, bigger than the whole family's put together.

MOTHER: If you do that (*fiddle with your widdler*) I
shall send for the doctor to cut off your widdler, and
then what will you widdle with?
HANS: With my bottom. (*Indicates widdler.*) Why don't
you put your finger there?
MOTHER: Because it's not proper.
HANS: (*Laughing.*) But it's great fun.

When asked later by father why he was laughing at his
sister Hanna's widdler, Hans replied 'Because her widdler's so lovely.' A sensible lad. On holiday among the
romantic mountain lakes he wanted to sleep with his
fourteen-year-old girl-friend Mariedl. The family had no
objections, but Freud sucked his teeth.

Freud was rightly proud at exposing through playful
Little Hans the sexuality of the sexually immature. But
as Hans' treatment was conducted, except for one consultation, between Freud and the father, suspicion must
fall upon parental obsession with the widdler. The widdler must have dominated family conversation as bor-
ingly as television today, when parents are equally nosy
and peppery about their children's widdlers, which are
now called their sex roles. Little Hans next encountered
Freud as an elegant twenty-year-old musician, but luckily had forgotten all about it.

The Rat Man served Emperor Franz Josef as an Army
officer. On manoeuvres in 1907, he heard in the mess
about a Chinese punishment, in which a pot of rats was
secured to the offender's bum, their only escape by
gnawing their way through the flesh and then emerging
from the anal exit. The rodents' instinct for anatomy so
obsessed the officer that he became confused and suici-
dal. Freud ascribed it to his exploring the genitalia of his
childhood governess. After a year, Freud cured the Rat
Man, just in time for him to be killed in World War One.

The Wolf Man kept dreaming that the tree outside his

bedroom window was crammed with wolves instead of birds. As reasonably as Little Red Riding-hood, he developed a phobia about wolves. Freud found that it was all through noticing his parents copulate in childhood. 'Yet Freud strangely ignored the Wolf Man's adult practice of anal intercourse,' murmurs a biographer. The Wolf Man was a rich Russian landowner who was visiting Vienna in 1914, became impoverished by the Revolution of 1917, and returned for more treatment in 1919, for which Freud had the decency not to charge.

The Wolf Man later blamed Freud for dissuading him from returning to Russia and reclaiming his riches from the Communists (Freud had psychological, not political, reasons for advising against this ridiculous risk), and got a job with a Viennese insurance company. The Wolf Man continued enjoying free psychological treatment even after World War Two, analysts from America seeking him in the spirit of tourists visiting the pyramids. Rightly so, because these cases stand in worthy magnificence in Freud's memory, however grotesquely they arise from the desert of unconsciousness.

'At the end of 1892,' revealed another of Freud's flocking biographers, 'he also failed with Miss Lucy R, an English governess who was suffering from general fatigue and exhibited the curious symptom of being haunted by the smell of burnt pudding.'

Tuesday, 6 September 1892

Berggasse, Vienna. A broad, complacent street, half a mile long, in north-west Vienna beyond the Schotten Ring. It runs from the Allgemeines Krankenhaus (where Ignaz Semmelweiss singlehandedly pole-axed childbed fever), with the Anatomical Institute (which caused the fever) standing on the corner, towards the Franz Josef

Quay against the Danube Canal. Number 19 is a heavy-fronted grey building of chiselled concrete, its hefty round-arched entrance, wide enough to accept a carriage, wearing as an afterthought a squashed pediment, and medalled with the Teutonic black-and-white number plate. To the right of the stolidly-carved oak front door, a shop-blind shades a butcher's window containing neatly parcelled veal and plump, albino Viennese sausages.

Standing on the tiled pavement is a pale-and-pink, perky-nosed English, even Reynoldsish, young woman in her mid-twenties, her brown hair piled high under a flat sepia straw hat, her slim form in brown cambric, tight-wristed with baggy sleeves, undecorated by brooch or bows from high neckband to the tips of her black boots. A brown knitted shawl is folded across her shoulders, she has brown cotton gloves, a small fringed russet handbag dangling from her elbow, and a tightly furled umbrella.

'*Guten Morgen! Mein Name ist* Miss Lucy Robinson,' she is informing the black-bombazined maid.

She is led inside, to a room between ground and first floor.

'*Er wird jeden Augenblick hier sein.*'

'*Danke!*'

Miss Lucy sits alone, straight-backed, hands atop brolly, on the edge of a comfortable couch which is covered to the floor with a densely patterned Persian rug, which climbs a yard up the plain wallpaper behind. There are two velvet cushions, a folded blanket, an untouched square pillow. Lots of small pictures in heavy frames – primitives, if you ask her – a scattered crowd of statuettes, ancient Chinese and Egyptian, they looked like. Tall windows upon a courtyard with three trees, and the inevitable Viennese ceramic stove in the corner. When Freud's sister Rosa later moved out, he could incorporate this early consulting-room into his eighteen-room flat upstairs. In 1895, Freud was on the phone. He made the address world renowned. He lived there until 4 June 1938.

Hurried steps downstairs. Appearance of a plumpish, amicable, hardly middle-aged-looking man in a dark suit and a pale tie, with floppy black hair and a beautiful beard (he went to the barber's daily). Everyone overlooks that even Freud was young once.

'Shall I take *der Regenschirm? Es ist schöns Wetter*. I have never before had a patient from England, Miss Robinson,' Freud began apologetically, accepting the umbrella. 'It is a country which I greatly admire. My son who was born last year I named Oliver, after Cromwell, your great Lord Chancellor until 1688.'

'Lord Protector,' she corrected, as though helping a slow child over a historical style. 'The Restoration was in 1660. It was the Glorious Revolution in 1688.'

'Ah! Thank you. Why did you travel all this way from tranquil England to cosmopolitan Vienna to instruct Dr Schmitt's children?'

'It was the cosmopolitanism my father wished me to endure. He is the Reverend Horace Robinson, the vicar of Slaughter-on-the-Marsh in the Cotswolds. It is a charming village – the church, St Laurence's, is largely ninth century – but somewhat remote amid the wheat and potatoes. The nearest railway is at Birmingham.'

'The English countryside has a famous beauty,' he said politely. 'One has only to look at the paintings of Turner.'

'Constable. And I believe my father wished to thin out his unmarried daughters. He has seven.'

Interest was triggered on Freud's face. 'Did you experience any intense love for your father?'

'Yes. As a child.'

Freud nodded thoughtfully.

'He always let me have the top of his boiled egg at breakfast.'

'Would you lie on the couch?' Freud invited.

'*Das ist sehr freundlich von Ihnen.*'

'Please give me your hat . . . you may care to unbutton your boots. So . . .' Coming to business: 'You are always tired?'

'I believe I simply do not get enough sleep,' Miss Lucy asserted calmly, reclining. 'The house is capacious and airy – the nursery food, I would add, is excellent – but my room overlooks the *Bahnhof*. Naturally, I sleep with the windows open. For the fresh air.'

Freud sat on a green velvet armchair which stood with a velvet-cushioned footstool behind the head of the couch. 'You are not suffering, perhaps, from the chlorosis? That makes so many young women tired.'

'Dr Schmitt excludes the chlorosis. He was insistent that I should consult you.'

'He is one of my enthusiasts,' said Freud fondly. 'We studied together at the Salpêtrière Hospital in Paris, six or seven years ago, under the famous Dr Charcot.'

'I know. Dr Schmitt often tells over meals how you both watched Dr Charcot hypnotise a young lady who was paralysed, and the great French doctor instantly cured her. The cause of her disability fascinates me. Her engagement to a man she did not love.'

Freud nodded briskly.

'Dr Schmitt finishes the story by declaring that this case revealed to you, in a thunderflash, the power of the unconscious mind.'

Freud smiled. 'He has a talent for exaggeration.'

'That is precisely what Dr Schmitt says about Dr Charcot.'

'Dr Schmitt also has a talent for cynicism. Such stories were going round Paris . . . But the *idea* which Dr Charcot transmitted to me was enough. The patient herself was but . . . what shall I say? An illustration in his textbook. *Das versteht sich,*' he added defensively.

Miss Lucy pursed her lips. 'I have thought about the notion, too. The unconscious mind.'

'It may help if you tell me,' he invited.

'It certainly never occupied any conscious thought in my home,' she instructed him. 'My father would have become extremely muddled had anyone mentioned it. Even "the will" and "the conscience" he was reluctant to discuss. Not that anyone at Slaughter-in-the-Marsh intruded with them often. In an English country parish, the vicar needs be a practical man. The poor, the sick and the sinners are more solidly identifiable.' She drew a breath. 'I saw the mind as a clock.'

Freud raised his eyebrows.

'A Swiss cuckoo-clock. We glance at the hands without pondering, we look up when the cuckoo bursts noisily into song, but everything we see or hear of the clock is powered by a strong, entirely hidden spring. That strikes *me* as the working of the unconscious mind.'

'Well! And you, Miss Robinson, have your charming national talent for understatement. I suppose it's a sound if simple comparison,' he conceded courteously. 'Now, this smell of burnt pudding.' He decided it desirable to come to the point. 'What sort of pudding?'

'Sometimes burnt rice pudding. Sometimes burnt bread-and-butter pudding – that is a nursery pudding we take in England, doctor, it is most agreeable. Sometimes burnt suet-pudding. Or jam roly-poly.'

'It haunts your nights?' Freud sat with a sheaf of paper. 'I should like to hear of your dreams.'

'My dreams?' She twisted her head to him. 'But they fly forgotten, just as time like an ever-rolling stream bears all its sons away.'

'Shakespeare,' he nodded.

'Hymns. Ancient and Modern.'

'Thank you. Miss Robinson, will you please write all your future dreams down for me, on waking up in the morning?'

'If you wish. I must remember a notebook and sharpened pencil tonight on my bed-table.' She crossed her hands gently across her stomach, with her gloves neatly folded across her handbag at her side. 'Dr Schmitt said you would be raising matters that, in different company, would be of extraordinary indelicacy. The warning seemed to give him amusement.'

'Should I say, the great majority of severe neuroses in women have their origin in the marriage bed?' He added with pointed off-handedness: 'An argument I shall be advancing in my *Studies on Hysteria*, to be published next year.'

'The marriage bed? Which I am as unlikely to sound as the bed of the ocean.'

Freud complimented her: 'Modesty is a charming attribute in any bride.'

'There is no modesty about it. There is nothing like being the member of a large family, which is sustained by the world spiritual, to induce a pressing temporal reality. A governess with no money of her own is as unmarriageable as a lame filly is unmountable.'

He protested amiably: 'But surely in England a "good family" is an inestimable dowry? You need only read the works of Charles Thackeray.'

'William Makepeace. No. A vicar's daughter is not socially excitable to the moneyed class. It is a universally accepted article of faith that the clergy may be openheartedly invited to tea, which may be delicious, with cucumber sandwiches and Dundee cake, but never to the socially equating ceremony of dinner.'

'I will take it you are *virgo intacta*.'

'Oh, dear me, no. If God makes a gift which the whole of mankind wishes to use eagerly – sometimes with quite alarming fervour – it would be irreligious and, worse, stupid, not to use it. You would not mute the morning birdsong with earplugs, not paint your windows black against the sunlight, nor abstain nervously from the delicious strawberries and cream which God sends each summer?'

Freud nodded solemnly. '*Das versteht sich von selbst.* The pleasure principle.'

'Why make a principle of pleasure?' she asked, puzzled. 'It is delightful enough on its own. And there is so little of it.'

An instructive idea occurred to him. 'Should I put it, sexuality is a powerful alloy, giving tension to that tight-wound, relentlessly unwinding spring which drives your cuckoo-clock. An alloy we name libido.'

'It sounds like a children's game.'

'I can assure you that children, and even babies, know how to play it.'

Miss Lucy continued calmly: 'In England, I have a gentleman friend. Yes, Captain Bracewell-Gregory. Of the Light Dragoons. He spotted me from his horse as I was going to church, and henceforth attended Matins every Sunday, in the front pew and singing extremely loudly. My father could hardly help noticing him, and later in conversation got the impression that Captain Bracewell-Gregory was a deeply religious man, and let him take me out on picnics.'

Freud thoughtfully stroked his scented beard. '*Ich habe mich entschlossen.* We are a case of penis envy.'

Miss Lucy frowned faintly. 'I don't think I *envied* Captain Bracewell-Gregory's penis. Mind you, I admit I considered it unfairly convenient for him on our delight-ful picnics, just standing up behind a tree when I was obliged to sit on my heels among the ferns. But I thought it a rather awkward organ to possess, and as for the appendages, why, it was like having a pawnbroker's sign dangling down your underwear. No, I didn't envy it at all,' she enlightened him firmly.

'Your trouble may equally well be an expression of the Oedipus complex,' Freud countered, making a note with his fountain-pen.

'I do not understand what you mean. At a dame-school you cannot expect education in the classics.'

'In a nutshell, as you so neatly say in England, every little boy has the desire to marry his mother. To achieve which he must obviously first kill his father. He develops fear that his father wishes to avoid both predicaments by castrating his son. It is equally applicable to females, when it is named the Electra complex. *Electra* was a play by Sophocles, a Greek writer of whom you may have heard. These impulses, of course, rage like the fires of our world, deep below the peaceful and unaware surface,' he clarified.

'I should hope so! Carving the Sunday joint is quite enough swordplay for any *pater familias*.'

'You will realise, we all of us have in our minds the Ego restraining the dark desires of the Id.'

'Like Papa and us daughters.'

'The Ego being wholly controlled by the Super Ego.'

'Like Mama.'

Freud rose. 'We shall have another consultation next month. After your dreams. There is a reason hidden deep in the mind for your smell of burnt pudding, Miss Robinson. Just as there must have been for King Alfred burning the cakes.'

'If you say so, I am sure there was an unconscious reason even for Napoleon burning Moscow,' she said graciously, sitting up and reaching for her boots.

'*Wie ist heute das Wetter?* I have not been out this morning.'

'Distinctly chilly. Shall I lie on the couch? Here are my dreams.' Miss Lucy took from her handbag a scroll of foolscap tied with yellow ribbon. 'I copied out my pencilled notes every morning while the children were completing their writing exercises.'

She pulled off her boots. Freud sat on the velvet chair, shuffling the foolscap pages. They were covered with copperplate and underlined regularly in red. 'You dreamt of ascending in a balloon!' he noticed, with suppressed excitement. 'I expect you often dream of flying? Such dreams are common, and are to be interpreted as expressions of sexual arousal.'

'Forgive me if I do not follow you, doctor.'

'Well, many women dream of balloons rising through the sky,' he explained. 'Through the remarkable property of the male sexual organ to rise up, in singular defiance of the laws of gravity.'

'How strange you should say so,' she agreed, settling comfortably on the couch. 'I made exactly the point to Captain Bracewell-Gregory, of the Light Dragoons, on one of our picnics. He explained, much amused, that his Hampton – '

'Hampton?'

'Hampton Wick. A district in London. On the Thames, near Hampton Court.'

Freud remained puzzled.

'It rhymes with "prick", a term used by Captain Bracewell-Gregory's soldiers to describe the organ you mention. Such rhyming is common among ordinary people. To "flash one's Hampton", I understand, is when they expose it to one of the other sex, uninvited. Captain Bracewell-Gregory opined that the Hampton elevated like an artillery piece taking aim, once it saw the target. He made a droll remark of its being mounted on ball-bearings.'

'*Verzeihen Sie!* I have lit a cigar. I often forget, when I have patients.'

'Please do. I fancy my dream was more likely occasioned by Dr Schmitt returning late from a medical dinner and attempting to fly up the staircase.'

Freud sighed. 'He is a good fellow, but he is no enemy of the bottle. For myself,' he admitted virtuously, 'I have the fear as your Duke of Clarence of drowning in a butt of sherry.'

'Malmsey.' Miss Lucy twiddled her toes in her white cotton stockings. 'You would seem to lay undue emphasis on the appurtenances of sexual union,' she told him firmly. 'My father had us all read Lord Chesterfield's *Letters to his Son*, from whom I recall a remark elsewhere, in that context: "The pleasure is momentary, the position ridiculous, and the expense damnable." '

'*Richtig!* You dream that I am pointing your umbrella at you,' Freud continued, finger on foolscap. 'That is my penis. So is the hammer you dream I hold in my other hand, the fountains you dream that I approach you among, the fish that you dream to be leaping from them. You are holding a bucket and leaving the door of a spacious church, both of which are your own genitalia.'

'I cannot answer for you, doctor, but speaking for my own appurtenances I fail to see any resemblance.'

'Pistols are penises, so are rifles, swords, lances, pencils and pens,' Freud told her ardently, his pen quivering vertical. 'Cupboards, ovens, ships, snails, anything hollow are the *muliebria*,' he continued, controlling with difficulty the enthusiasm for his own ideas. 'Your dreams, Miss Robinson, are the joyous fulfilment of your sexual longings, of your frustrated urges of the day. These desires always appear in your dreams, but always in disguise.'

'But surely, that occurred to Johann Strauss twenty years ago?'

'*Wie bitte?*' asked Freud shortly.

'For Frau Schmitt's birthday, Dr Schmitt kindly invited me to accompany them to the Theater an der Wien for a performance of *Die Fledermaus*. I paid close attention, having only once before been to the opera, to see Mr Gilbert's *Gondoliers* at the Savoy Theatre in London, which was most amusing. In *Die Fledermaus*, at Prince Orlofsky's ball in the Second Act, I remember particularly that the hero, the handsome Herr von Eisenstein, and his beautiful wife Rosalinde, and her flirtatious maid Adele, all caper about most enjoyably. But all are masked! You see, doctor,' she ended triumphantly, 'each is totally unaware of the other's identity, however improbable it may seem. This is surely exactly as you are saying that our thoughts behave in our dreams?'

'Possibly,' said Freud brusquely.

'The music was so catchy. Dr Schmitt seems quite to like my singing it, standing beside him while he plays the piano.'

'At our first consultation, you forgot your handbag.'

She nodded. 'Indeed. I had to return all the way from Währinger Strasse, with the horses of my bus already approaching round the corner.'

'That was a sexual proposition towards me.'

She raised her delicate eyebrows. 'Then it must have been a singularly absent-minded one.'

'It cannot be interpreted otherwise,' Freud informed her confidently. 'You have transferred an emotional dependence from your father to myself. You are in love with me.'

'All of which is the cause of my smell of burnt pudding?'

'Undoubtedly.'

'Perhaps I should have mentioned earlier, but I was so eager to talk of my dreams – my sisters and I discuss our dreams over breakfast, it is remarkable how one's own dreams are fascinating, while those of others are literally unbelievably boring, though I suppose dreams to you are all in the day's work, like coughs and cuts to other doctors – I was going to tell you, that Frau Schmitt's cook has secretly been attempting to perfect a *sachertorte* for the doctor's own birthday, so far without success, and has been burning the evidence in the backyard under my window after the family was in bed.'

Silence.

'From my assessment of your personality, Miss Robinson, I think you have discovered the perfectly correct diagnosis of your case,' he conceded, with unconscious relief.

'Thank you, Dr Freud,' she said gratefully, rising from the couch. 'I have much enjoyed pouring out so many things to you, that I should otherwise have kept hidden from the world. Captain Bracewell-Gregory of the Light Dragoons, for instance. It has made me feel very much better, mentally and even physically. And your theories about the unconscious mind and the sexual performance are perfectly fascinating. I am sure if you persist with such chats you will become much sought-after and quite famous. *Auf Wiedersehen!*'

Freud's Ghost

Everyone has heard of Freud, as of God. His word, which was expressed in some three million of them, now lies as dusty unconsulted files in the basement of psychiatry. The concoction of his theories was surely glory enough. He modestly, and rightly, quoted fellow Viennese

Christian Friedrich Hebbel, the gloomy dramatist of the mid-nineteenth century, saying that he had himself 'Disturbed the sleep of the world'. And the world's sleepily opening eye discovered that there was much more in man than met it. Or was Freud only the Jules Verne of twenty thousand leagues under the consciousness?

Freud's shadow fell shorter as the sexual sky brightened. The horrifying secrets of his couch are tonight's television programmes. He had his dissidents. Carl Gustav Jung (1875–1961) of Zurich broke away in 1911 and watered down the libido. Viennese Alfred Adler (1870–1937) felt that all small boys did not really want to have sex with their mothers. Henry Havelock Ellis (1859–1939) from Croydon reclassified Freud as an artist, not a scientist. Jolly, vain Wilhelm Stekel (1868–1940) cheerfully expressed his own relationship to Freud as: 'A dwarf on the shoulder of a giant can see further than the giant himself.' About which, Freud observed: 'That may be true, but a louse on the head of an astronomer does not.'

Freud's teaching was busily propagated by his phantoms, richly walking the dreams of the world, particularly American. Analysts continue to unburden life's strugglers and stragglers of their elaborately packaged troubles, towards which family and friends might possibly express shock, but certainly feel boredom. Psychoanalysis has an oddity: it is the only cure for any condition to be attempted by talking about it. Which has one increasingly prized advantage in medicine: no side-effects.

Man's Unconquerable Mind

Freud accelerated one wickedly lazy transformation in medicine, of madness into illness. Before the nineteenth century, the insane had nothing to lose but their chains. The worst were dangerous and terrifying, the best harmless but irritating, the most resented those in your own family. Madmen and madwomen were sagaciously kept shackled, two of them in the Bicêtre Hospital in Paris for forty years, until 24 May 1798. Then Philippe Pinel (1745–1826) arrived to strike the links from all forty-nine inmates, and carry them off to equally intelligent physicians among his friends. Pinel had been urging this liberation since 1792, when Dr Guillotin's busy instrument started cropping Paris. The National Assembly participated in his compassion, but in such excitable times Pinel was attacked by an alarmed mob, until the freed monsters themselves appeared for his rescue.

Eponymous 'Bedlam', to which Hogarth's Rake finally progressed, was the Hospital of St Mary of Bethlehem, founded by the Sheriff of London in 1247 as a stopover for bishops and canons. By 1402 it was housing lunatics in Bishopsgate, up from the Tower. After the dissolution of the monasteries, Henry VIII presented it in 1547 to the City of London as a madhouse. In 1675 it was rebuilt beside London Wall and the public charged to view the lunatics, like the Zoo. This went on till 1815. The same facility was offered in 1784 by the 'Lunatics' Tower' in Vienna.

Yorkshire tea and coffee merchant and Quaker William Tuke (1732–1822) in 1796 rescued the local mad into the York Retreat. There were no chains, no 'strait-waistcoats, handcuffs, leg-locks, various coarse devices of leather and iron, including gags and screws, to force open the mouths of unhappy patients who were unwilling or even unable to take food'. It was the first 'asylum': a lovely Greek word, a sanctuary, an inviolable place of refuge, such a pity it shudders with derogatory overtones like 'suburbia'.

The Victorians scattered asylums round the countryside in lofty red-brick and slate, like the new universities. The sprawling buildings enjoyed sweeping views, extensive vegetable gardens, vast kitchens, oversized laundries and endless corridors, all providing diverting but simple work for the inmates. The doors were kept locked, the windows opened but two inches, the lavatory chains were enclosed in piping to forestall hanging, the males seldom saw the females, and thus humans passed their deranged lives, comfortably camouflaged from public view.

Luckily, asylums offered little medical treatment. The efficiency of traditional opium, camphor, belladonna and vinegar, of the mustard or Spanish fly plasters to the head, of the enemas, emetics, and cold douches was beginning to incur doubt. In 1935, drugs induced convulsions in schizophrenics, in the muddled belief that schizophrenia and epilepsy could not cohabit the same brain. 'ECT' – electroconvulsion therapy – was later applied to depressives, less upsettingly under anaesthesia during World War Two; even less so, when anaesthetists adopted the paralytic poison curare, so that convulsion therapy could be effectively given without the convulsions.

After the war come the antidepressant drugs, anxiolytics, hypnotics, powerful tranquillizers for schizophrenia, and lithium salts to stabilise manic-depressives. A population which would indignantly claim to be perfectly sane now swallows psychotropic drugs as blithely as sprinkling sugar on its cornflakes. The asylums became mental hospitals, which then became hospitals, and then the doors were flung wide to release the drugged patients into the community, which is the hard world.

Our murderous and dangerous lunatics are secured in mental prisons. The harmless ones are secreted away in psychiatric wards. The rest may sleep in the streets, for all we care. Sane thinking about insanity has neatly returned to 1547.

ELEVEN

Scholars, Truants and Teachers' Pets

That's what makes the medical student the most disgusting figure in modern civilisation. No veneration, no manners –

George Bernard Shaw,
The Doctor's Dilemma.

Pity as a Motive

Attend to Charles Dickens:

> 'Nothing like dissecting, to give one an appetite,' said Mr Bob Sawyer, looking round the table.
> Mr Pickwick slightly shuddered.
> 'Bye the bye, Bob,' said Mr Allen, 'have you finished that leg yet?'
> 'Nearly,' replied Sawyer, helping himself to half a

fowl as he spoke. 'It's a very muscular one for a child's.'

'Is it?' inquired Mr Allen, carelessly.

'Very,' said Bob Sawyer, with his mouth full.

'I've put my name down for an arm, at our place,' said Mr Allen. 'We're clubbing for a subject, and the list is nearly full, only we can't get hold of any fellow that wants a head. I wish you'd take it.'

'No,' replied Bob Sawyer; 'can't afford expensive luxuries.'

'Nonsense!' said Allen.

'Can't indeed,' rejoined Bob Sawyer. 'I wouldn't mind a brain, but I couldn't stand a whole head.'

'Hush, hush, gentlemen, pray,' said Mr Pickwick, 'I hear the ladies.'

Dear medical students! Dear Dickens! At their own age, how light-handedly you grasped their alarming qualities. Dr John Brown (1810–82) of Edinburgh pinned the paradox fourteen years later:

> Don't think medical students heartless; they are neither better nor worse than you or I: they get over their professional horrors, and into their proper work; and in them pity – as an *emotion*, ending in itself or at best in tears and a long drawn breath, lessens, while pity, as a *motive*, is quickened, and gains power and purpose. It is well for poor human nature that it is so.

When life and death will become your bread-and-butter, it is reasonable to view them as prosaically as the hospital sandwiches.

Rising Above It

Four medical scholars:

– Sir Thomas Browne (1605–82) was far too intelligent to be a GP in Norwich, but he stayed in that agreeable place with the Norman cathedral for forty-six years, because he preferred a quiet life pottering inquisitively amid the local butterflies and relics and wondering about death and having ten children. To pass the time he wrote *Religio Medici*, which in 1642 examined the straining yoke of science and religion so sensibly that three years later it made the Roman Catholic Church's *Index of Prohibited Books*.

'I borrow not the rules of my Religion from Rome or Geneva, but the dictates of my own reason,' Browne said primly. He shared any East Anglian farmer's disbelief in forbidden fruit: 'In the same Chapter when GOD forbids it, 'tis positively said, the plants of the field were not yet grown, *for* GOD *had not caus'd it to rain upon the earth.*' Sir Thomas shook his head over Judgment Day, which seemed to him an extension of Norwich Assizes. When he was knighted, Charles II had to go to Norwich to do it.

When the Funerall pyre was out, and the last valediction over, and men took a lasting adieu of their interred Friends, 'Who knows the fate of his bones?' Sir Thomas asked in *Urn Burial*. His own bones were fated in 1840 to lose their skull, which remained on show in the Norfolk and Norwich Hospital until 1922. He had a hate of witchcraft, and in 1664 temporarily left Norwich to get Amy Duny and Rose Cullender hanged for it down the road at Bury St Edmunds.

– Oliver Wendell Holmes (1809–94) was *The Autocrat of the Breakfast-table* and Professor of Anatomy at Harvard for thirty-five years. In 1843, he suggested that fatal puerperal fever was contagious, and avoidable by the attending doctor washing his hands and changing his clothes. This was four years before Ignaz Semmelweiss said the same thing in Vienna. In Boston, such gratuitous criticism of personal hygiene caused outrage. A long life allowed the Autocrat to proclaim victoriously, after Pasteur and Koch: 'a little army of microbes was marched up to support my position.'

When William Morton gave birth in Boston to ether, the Autocrat bustled over the christening:

Everybody wants to have a hand in a great discovery. All I will do is to give you a hint or two, as to names ... the state should, I think, be called 'Anaesthesia'. This signifies insensibility, more particularly to objects of touch.

Luckily discarding antineuric, neuro-lepsia and neuro-etasis, Holmes rightly foresaw that 'anaesthesia' would 'be repeated by the tongues of every civilised race of mankind'. After Queen Victoria inhaled chloroform for the birth of Prince Leopold, it became in London a fashionable christian name for baby girls. Twenty years later: 'My lord, may I introduce your dinner partner? My daughter Anaesthesia.'

– Sir William Osler Bt (1849–1919) from Bond Head, Ontario, was successively Professor of Medicine at Montreal (aged twenty-five), Philadelphia, Baltimore and Oxford. He was blithe and benign, handsomely walrus-moustached, the perceiver of Osler's nodes (on the fingertips in heart infections), and the great-grandson-in-law of Paul Revere. He exhibited such enthusiasm for his profession that 'He went into the post-mortem room with the joyous demeanour of the youthful Sophocles leading the chorus of victory after the battle of Salamis,' which must have been trying. A besought teacher and prolific expounder (730 books and scientific papers), Sir William was the Francis Bacon of the medical profession (the modifying effect of the adjective is considerable, as Thomas Mann remarked when Goethe was described as the German Voltaire).

In 1900, Osler advised that all persons of sixty should be painlessly and unfussily exterminated. This pronouncement from Baltimore of so godlike a physician induced fits in the American press. Such a convenience for mankind had already been suggested by Anthony Trollope's novel *The Fixed Period*, published in the year of Trollope's death, 1882 (the story was set in 1980, you ended with a dose of morphine, then your veins were cut open while relaxing in a warm bath, it all happened in New Zealand, anyway).

The pair were short-sighted prophets. It is unnecessary to specify that the world has too many people, and they all want to park their cars. The globe's population is exploding by 250,000 babies a day, which by the year 2000 will add to our present 5.3 billion yet another billion, or one China. During the coming century global population will treble, or only double if we are lucky. Meanwhile, the more sparingly reproductive people of the northern hemisphere will live longer and longer, through the familiar miracles of modern medicine, but in ever-increasing decrepitude. It cannot be distant before Zimmer walking-frames will be clamped on yellow lines or carted away to pounds.

The stability of civilisation demands a chain of Terminal Inns, remote in delightful scenery like the TB sanatoriums of the 1930s, with supreme dining, floorshows and dancing, everything free including drinks, gambling chips and sex (where achievable), until one night, with cyanide gas in the air-conditioning, each inmate is softly and suddenly vanished away, as the over-venturesome Baker hunting the Snark. It is foreshadowed by a Society for the Right to Die in the United States, though admittedly they take death there unnecessarily seriously.

The ardour of both Trollope's characters and of Sir William for the idea waned in synchrony with their fifth decade.

– John Locke (1632–1704), was a doctor sixteen years before *An Essay Concerning Human Understanding*.

The medical profession enjoys a historical attraction towards the profession of letters, which never calls you out at night, nor even in inclement weather, and you can get as drunk as you like at lunchtime. Doctor-novelists bulk the stable fodder of the bookshelves: François Rabelais (c 1495–1553), Conan Doyle, de Vere ('Blue Lagoon') Stacpoole (1863–1951), Francis Brett Young (1884–1954), A. J. Cronin (1896–1981), Somerset Maugham. They are surprisingly outnumbered by Keats, Robert Bridges (1844–1930), Thomas Campion (1567–1620), Abraham Cowley (1618–16<7), George Crabbe (1754–1832), Schiller (1759–1805) and other medical poets: perhaps an intense youthful fascination with human beings and eternity is thought better directed to the financially less risky occupation of medicine.

Anton Chekhov (1860–1904), who found enjoyably that 'the Stage is a noisy, flashy, and insolent mistress', was flattered by psychiatric consultant to the media Anthony Clare (b 1942) as: 'The only one who seemed able to use the material of medicine and really elevate it to the levels of high art. Otherwise medicine usually breeds middle-rank writers.' Osborne Henry Mavor (1888–1951), Professor of Medicine at Glasgow, wrote as James Bridie witty, talkative, mildly Chekhovian plays like *The Anatomist* (about Robert Knox and Burke and Hare), and a definitive scientific paper on that anatomical hub *The Umbilicus*, which he discovered could get eight diseases.

Dr Peter Mark Roget (1779–1869) founded Manchester medical school and London University, investigated London's water supply, invented the logo-logarithmic slide-rule, wrote on physiology and theology, and in 1852 produced Roget's *Thesaurus*. He was a polymath, polyhistor, pantologist, encyclopaedist, prodigy of learning, mine of information, walking encyclopaedia, talking dictionary. Dr Samuel Smiles (1812–1904) extended this helpful simile service with *Self Help*. Dr Thomas Bowdler (1754–1825) of Edinburgh bowdlerised Shakespeare.

Individualists

Yorkshire surgical magnifico Lord Moynihan (1865–1936) gave the Linacre Lecture at Cambridge in May 1936 on 'Truants'. Moynihan was a champion operator, when often only the surgeon's skill separated the patient's life and death. 'There is nothing in the craft of any art so exquisitely beautiful that it can surpass that shown by the skilful master of surgery,' he said, throwing an interesting challenge to the Royal Ballet. He named 'Moynihan's Gutter' inside the abdomen, and Moynihan's gall-bladder forceps. His father was a sergeant who won the VC in the Crimea.

Fifteen doctors who found better things to do:

— Andrew Boorde (?1490–1549) wrote *Tom Thumb*, studied medicine in Montpellier, became a Carthusian monk, then suffragan bishop of Chichester in 1521. The original Merry Andrew, he anticipated modern habits by making funny after-feast speeches at fairs, by writing a phrase-book in Cornish, Welsh, Castilian, Dutch and Gypsy, and through *The Breviarie of Health* giving advice on dieting, house-buying, personal finance, fashions, sex, jogging and sleep. He was a secret agent of Thomas Cromwell, sent to France and Spain in 1535 to find how people were feeling about Henry VIII. He was uncomfortable in Glasgow, where he briefly practised: 'Trust yow no Skott, for they wyll yowse flatterying wordes, and all ys falshode.' Died in jail.

— Georges Benjamin Clemenceau (1841–1929) practised in Montmartre, before teaching French to schoolgirls in Stratford, Connecticut, and becoming Prime Minister and Minister of War in Paris in 1917.
— Henry Faulds (1844–1930) from Glasgow, for ten years ran the Tsukiji Hospital, Tokyo, where he conceived fingerprints. The first ever were impressed in 1880, on ten finger-outlines produced by Japanese engravers. What would his contemporary Sir Arthur Conan Doyle have done without him?
— Richard Jordan Gatling (1818–1903) came from North Carolina and invented the Gatling gun, which fired 350 shots a minute.
— William Gilbert Grace (1848–1915) of Gloucestershire and England requires no identification in any English book.
— Joseph Ignace Guillotin (1738–1814) was elected to *L'Assemblé nationale* in 1789, where he originated history's most impressive practical demonstration of democracy: that the common people could be beheaded like the aristocracy. The ordinary man had formerly been merely hanged. Dr Guillotin's invention could also substitute for cruel punishments like the tearing apart by four horses, when the executioner often needed to slice into the prisoner's arm and leg joints when the poor beasts became tired.

Guillotin was a busybody do-gooder, who sat on Louis XVI's Commission investigating Anton Mesmer's animal magnetics, and was an expert on ventilation. He conceived the guillotine, but it was designed by his surgical colleague Antoine Louis (1723–92), discoverer of the angle of Louis, which you can feel an inch down your breastbone. The first one was built by a German harpsichord maker, Tobias Schmidt. Its terminology enjoys the casual French elegance of that of skiing: the *mouton*, the 35 kilogram weight that speeds the downward blade, the *déclic* which the *bourreau* presses to apply it to the patient, who is pushed standing up against the *bascule*, which instantly see-saws him horizontal, for his neck to be encircled in the wooden *lunette*. His head is then steadied by the hair, or in cases of baldness the ears, by *le photographe*, lurking beyond a facing blood-proof screen. Had the guillotine taken on in England – one was decapitating busily in Halifax under Edward III – this crouching member of the execution team would inevitably be 'the wicket-keeper'.

Dr Guillotin's first operation was on 25 April 1792, in the Place de Grève, but he went private in 1939. The prisoner never knew the date, except that he could not become headless on Sunday or *jours fériés*. Then, in the darkest hour, bootless warders approached softly to unlock the door, to wake him and gave him a glass of rum and a cigarette and his civilian clothes back, including his hat. As Dr Guillotine obtained in a steely flash not one patient, but two, the head, perfectly nourished by the final thumping heartbeat, possibly continued to keep abreast of events. Charlotte Corday is famed for her post-mortem blushes, and several doctors have shouted at severed heads with encouraging response.

At 5.30 on a June morning in 1905, the condemned head fell neatly on its severed stump upright at a doctor's feet. Eyelids and lips continued blinking and pursing for some seconds. Then, on the doctor's calling the head's name, the eyelids slowly lifted 'such as happens in everyday life, with people awakened or torn from their thoughts', and its eyes fixed and focused on his own. The *croissants* afterwards would have been munched thoughtfully. Dr Guillotin died at home from a carbuncle.

– Sir Goldsworthy Gurney (1793–1875) was a Cornish surgeon so ingenious that he invented limelight, the oxyhydrogen blowpipe, a piano which played on musical glasses, the jet-propelled steamboat, the 1829 steam carriage in which he averaged 15 mph from London to Bath and back, an extinguisher for fires down coal mines, a signalling lamp, a way for seamen to identify lighthouses, and the Gurney Stove to warm up the House of Commons.

– Sir Leander Starr Jameson Bt (1853–1917) lies in the Matopo Hills overlooking Bulawayo from the south, near his close friend Cecil Rhodes, who got him out to run Rhodesia. On 29 December 1895 'Dr Jim' led his raid into the Transvaal, to liberate the British who had crowded to get at the gold and diamonds, and to whom the Boers were being beastly. This collapsed on New Year's Day.

– David Kinloch (1559–1617), obstetrician and poet, travelling from Dundee, was arrested by the Spanish Inquisition and sentenced to burning alive. This became postponed because the Grand Inquisitor fell ill. Kinloch sent a note by a black cat that he was a doctor, and could he help? He cured the Grand Inquisitor, and anointed with his gratitude went home to Scotland. Well, that is what it says in the *British Medical Journal* of 1 May 1926.

– The Rev Francis Thomas McDougall (1817–86), a surgeon, rowed for Oxford, became Bishop of Sarawak, and wrote with keen appreciation to *The Times*, after repelling an attack by Chinese pirates in 1862, about his London-made double-barrelled breechloader. It 'proved itself a most deadly weapon from its true shooting, certainty, and rapidity of fire. It never missed fire in 80 rounds, and I believe it would have fired 80 more with like effect'. This testimonial did not go over well with the ecclesiastical establishment, surveying its calm lawns, peaceful tea-tables and humane principles at home.

– Jean Paul Marat (1743–93), stabbed in his bath by Charlotte Corday, was MD St Andrews, Scotland. He was in the bath to relieve the itch of his eczema.

– Francis Moore (1657–1715), physician at Lambeth, London, in 1701 founded *Old Moore's Almanac*.

– James Parkinson (1755–1824) was accused of plotting to assassinate George III with a poisoned dart from a popgun at the theatre. His is the name of Parkinson's disease.

- James Startin (1806–72), a London dermatologist, discovered a cheap and efficient way to stiffen felt hats.
- Sir Charles Wyndham (1841–1919) from Liverpool, one of Lincoln's surgeons in the Civil War, returned to England and went on the stage. He is memorialised by Wyndham's theatre in the West End, though his real name was Culverwell. He was knighted by Edward VII in 1902, when both doctors and actors were being doubtfully awarded the respectability to trespass on these chivalrous preserves.

And five who distinguished themselves more than in medicine, where they failed to qualify:

- Armenian *émigré* Michael Arlen (1895–1956) of 1924's fashionable novel *The Green Hat*, studied medicine at Edinburgh. He was 'more brilliantine than brilliant', according to *The Times*.
- Hector Berlioz (1803–69), a Grenoble doctor's romantic son who infuriated his father by detesting medicine.
- Johann Wolfgang Goethe (1749–1832) drifted away from medical lectures in Strasburg, but in 1786 made a useful discovery of the intermaxillary bone in the upper jaw.
- Christopher Isherwood (1904–86) was a medical student at King's College, London, 1928–29.
- Cecil Scott Forester (1899–1966) was a student at Guy's Hospital, but launched Hornblower.

Bad Boys

Twelve medical pirates billowed through the seventeenth and eighteenth centuries. The most successful in both occupations was Thomas Dover (1660–1742). He was a man of such terrifying temper, that he could be relied upon never to attract sufficient subordinates to scuttle away with the loot. In 1709, as captain of the *Duke*, a year out of Bristol with the *Duchess*, Dover sacked Guayaquil in Peru, and cured 172 out of 180 of his crew of the plague by bleeding them from both arms until they fainted. Homeward bound, he rescued Alexander Selkirk (Robinson Crusoe) from the island of Juan Fernandez, then resumed his Bristol practice, obesely rich.

Like all physicians he had a favourite cure, which only fortunate patients matched with their disease. This was mercury, so he was renowned as 'The Quicksilver Doctor'. He invented Dover's powder, a cough-mixture of opium and the Brazilian root ipecacuanha, which flatteringly survived in British pharmacy until the age of penicillin. Dover was a pirate in the honourable Drake tradition. We are a nation of successful pirates, whose booty, the British Empire, survived for the same time as Dover's powder.

Medical murderers are memorable through their lurid incompetence. Dr Crippen of Hilldrop Crescent in London in 1910 buried his wife in the cellar (apart from her head, which has not yet surfaced). Dr Buck Ruxton near Blackpool in 1935 cut up his wife and nursemaid in the bath, ascribing the blood which soaked his staircarpet, curtains, suit and their nighties, to cutting his hand on a tin-opener with a can of peaches. Dr Pritchard of Glasgow killed his wife and mother-in-law in 1865 with aconite, and signed their death certificates himself (as apoplexy and typhoid). Dr Palmer of Rugeley gave a horse-racing friend strychnine in 1855, then tried to pocket his stomach during the post-mortem. Dr Cream from Canada killed several London tarts in 1891 with strychnine, the showy way, with violent fits. Clearly, only a modest professional skill was necessary for all those doctors who got away with murder.

Céline (Dr Louis-Ferdinand Destouches, 1894–1961)
thought: 'The medical is an invidious profession. When
one's practice is among the rich one looks like a lackey,
and when it's among the poor like a thief.' People used
to being treated as somebody important have difficulty
adjusting themselves to becoming only some body. More
alarming, what a disaster for everybody else in their
incapacity, or unspeakably their death! Churchill forthrightly commanded both his doctors and his diseases to
implement his own ideas. He luckily had the sympathetic assistance of Lord ('Corkscrew Charlie') Moran
(1882–1977), a man comfortably appreciative of his own
importance.

Hitler's doctor was fat, bald Theo Morell (1886–1948),
who was elevated to become an unpopular member of
the Führer's entourage from being a fashionable Berlin
practitioner in dermatology, venereology and impotence,
which he treated with electric shocks. Every other day,
Hitler lowered his uniform trousers for Morell to inject
vitamins into the *Führerrumph*. The ceremony increased
during the war to Hitler dropping them five times daily.
From 1936, when Hitler reoccupied the Rhineland and
showed Europe that he meant business (pathetically
ineffectively), until 1945 when he shot himself, his bride,
and his dog, Morell secretly supplemented the vitamins
with hefty doses of amphetamine. This made his patient
'fresh', alert, active, and immediately ready for the day
. . . cheerful, talkative, physically active and tending to
stay awake long hours into the night.' Hitler got an extra
dose when bad news came in. All Churchill got was
whisky.

Bismarck's doctors needed respectfully to curb an
appetite that nightly guzzled caviar to raise a thirst for
mugs of powerful beer, without which he could not

sleep. Frederick the Great's doctors needed to instil in their patient an enthusiasm for dandelion juice, to replace his favourite lunch of spiced soup, Russian beef in brandy, Italian maize with garlic, and savoury eel-pie. Louis XIV's had to keep quiet His Majesty's clap. George III's doctors faced remedying his madness.

From 1765 to 1810 poor King George suffered five attacks of insanity – howling like a dog, excitable, consorting with the invisible dead, chasing the ladies-in-waiting – each one lasting six months, the last lingering until his death in 1820 aged eighty-two. The disease foreseeably had political complications, which were eventually treated with the Regency of George IV in 1811. The royal doctors treated the King the current way, respectfully wrapping him in straitjackets. It was a madness caused by porphyria, a metabolic disorder, like diabetes and gout. It was a chemical deranged, not a king. But porphyrin was not discovered in the blood until 1863.

Queen Victoria's personal physician was Sir James Reid Bt (1849–1923), a humdrum Aberdonian GP whom she had picked up at Balmoral, who resembled an Easter egg luxuriantly glued with whiskers. Reid had studied in Vienna, so he offered the attraction of speaking the late Prince Albert's German with the accent of her devoted Highland ghillie John Brown, also his patient (Brown was a martyr to the wee dram).

On Reid's appointment in 1881, the Queen was a fit, if overweight, sixty-two, with a touch of the rheumatics and the wind (she gobbled her food, and poured Scotch in her claret). Exercising royally the prerogative of hypochondria, at Balmoral, Windsor or Osborne she summoned her miserably paid doctor six times daily, she snatched him from his holidays, and she wrote to him reassuringly on his honeymoon: 'The bowels are acting fully.' Such intimacy was entirely constitutional, and assuredly regally relished. It created Reid the Queen's personal person.

Sir James could execute and exert breath-taking influence at Court. No British doctor was gonged without his nod. When Gladstone retired in 1894, the Queen had Reid push her favoured replacement, Lord Rosebery, instead of Sir William Harcourt, because 'of saving the Queen's health'. Reid was a snob in the workshop of snobbery. He considered a Knight Bachelor fit 'for all sorts of common fellows' and stuck out for a KCB, which was six rungs higher up the Order of Precedence, and which he got after lunch at Balmoral in 1895, with a claymore.

As the Queen's favourite entertainment was watching babies descending or souls ascending, Sir James was her natural companion at aristocratic childbeds and death-beds. He implemented her loving instructions for the funerals of her relations, housemaids, and dog. At her own funeral in 1901, Sir James was secretly charged to slip into her coffined left hand the eighteen-year dead John Brown's photo, and a lock of his hair. Sir James had just then been able to diagnose that his royal patient had a hernia and had long suffered from a badly prolapsed uterus. In his twenty years as Physician in Ordinary and Physician Extraordinary, he had never seen the Queen with any of her clothes off. I wonder if the same went for her Highland ghillie.

On the Monday of 20 January 1936, King George V was dying at Sandringham, where the clocks were always kept one hour fast (Edward VII had ordered it for the punctual muster for his shooting-parties twenty-five years earlier). The royal physician was Lord Dawson of Penn (1864–1945), who was charming, sensitive, genial, impatient, a euthanasia enthusiast, a practised courtier, a manipulative politician. He was familiar in the news-papers, the signer of bulletins suspended on Buckingham

Palace railings to inform a straining crowd of their rulers' precarious health, and he was honoured beyond his profession as a Privy Counsellor.

About him that evening gathered the Prince of Wales (by air), Cosmo Lang the snobbish Archbishop of Canterbury, and Ramsay MacDonald the fussing and flapping Prime Minister. At dinner, Dawson scribbled on the back of a menu card his immortal intimation of mortality: 'The King's life is moving peacefully towards its close.' (You cannot create that over the soup. Dawson undoubtedly coined and polished it while the royal patient upstairs was himself still chomping and quaffing.)

While this news impinged on the anxious country via the BBC wireless, the Prince of Wales, the Dukes of York and Kent, and the King's private secretary collected for a businesslike planning of the funeral. Once he had got rid of the Archbishop from the bedchamber, Dawson found himself alone with 'calm and kindly' Queen Mary and the jumpy Prince of Wales. It came out alarmingly fifty years later that they had already promised Dawson that he need'st not strive Officiously to keep alive the King. So at eleven o'clock, Dawson injected a hefty dose of morphine and cocaine into the King's distended jugular vein, which knocked him off at five minutes to midnight.

The King's deadline was *The Times'* deadline. Dawson wanted the fatal announcement dignified by *The Times*, the editor already warned by Lady Dawson to hold the middle (front) page, instead of by the parvenu wireless, which he may have felt already had enough out of him that crowded evening. The Prince of Wales became hysterical and kept embracing the Queen, until succeeding to the Throne and immediately having the Sandringham clocks put back. Later that year Dawson was promoted in the Honours List, so setting a Viscountcy as the going rate for British regicide.

TWELVE

The Body Politic

Think of what our Nation stands for . . .
Democracy and proper drains.
John Betjeman,
'In Westminster Abbey'.

The Public Health

The Sanitary Conditions of the Labouring Population of Great Britain was published in 1842 by Sir Edwin Chadwick (1801–90), a Poor Law commissioner, a favourite of Jeremy ('the greatest happiness of the greatest number') Bentham, a lawyer and self-educated sanitary engineer, the creator of the Cawnpore drains in 1871, vocational busybody and browbeater and prototype enthusiast for the environment, which was still known as the heaven and the earth.

The labouring population's conditions were unlovely. The Romans had been a cleanly lot, the Tudors were into drains, but the sowers and spinners of our ancient rustic life 'blown through by the winds of heaven', had quit the pages of Thomas Hardy for those of Arnold Bennett. Half the nation had exchanged the squire's sway for the millowner's money, cramming itself into insanitary and worsening urban slums. The British death-rate, which had fallen joyfully between 1780 to 1810, hit a bleak plateau. Churchyards developed a turnover like prosperous inns. The bodies were dug up and tipped into pits, or (some said) crushed into bone-meal, then the room relet. Church crypts were packed like cadaverous sardines. Goaded by the local stink, Dr George ('Graveyard') Walker (1807–84) of Drury Lane remonstrated with his *Gatherings from Graveyards*, and stood accused of impiety. Chadwick backed him up, and in 1850 Parliament regulated what a cleric could lay down in his cellar.

Chadwick's *Sanitary Conditions* depicted poverty and disease as two sides of the same coin. But two sides of a coin are impossible to view together. Nothing was done about either misfortune. Luckily, there was a violent epidemic of cholera in 1847. Like Saul and David, typhus has slain his thousands, but cholera his ten thousands. Cholera killed 10,000 Londoners that summer, outshining the capital's usual hot weather epidemics. Five hundred died in the human rookeries of Soho, where the excrement of men and animals mixed on the rutted cobbles and the drains mixed with the drinking water. These were the 'cholera courts' of Miss Nightingale, who nursed the victims in nearby Middlesex Hospital. Miss Nightingale knew that cholera was caused by filth and cured by sanitation. She scorned as a passing superstition the notion of its spread by contagion (germs had not yet been invented). Like all her opinions, this was strong and enduring, even on the appearance of overwhelming evidence to the contrary.

The cholera so frightened Parliament, it passed the Public Health Act of 1848. This established a General Board of Health, containing Chadwick and Lord Shaftesbury (1801–85), the unflagging philanthropist and champion of lunatics, working women and juvenile chimney-sweeps. Shaftesbury was the founder (encouraged by Dickens) of the ragged schools, to corral wild children, have them clothed, shod, and instructed in the Bible, then deported to Australia.

The Board was a flop. A medical officer of health was appointed for London (trendy Liverpool already had one), but however forceful its recommendations there was no one to make them work. Except Sir Edwin Chadwick, who achieved a political notoriety unmatched until Edwina Currie laid an egg. *The Times* decided on 1 August 1854, about Chadwick's plan to pump into central London clean water from Surrey: 'We prefer to take our chances of cholera and the rest rather than be bullied into health.' *The Times* quoted itself on 15 June 1983, now writing about dieting to control our epidemic of coronary disease, adding ruefully: 'Perhaps too many of us retain the sentiments.' We do.

In 1853 Chadwick was fired, and five years later the Board of Health was absorbed by the Privy Council. In 1854, John Snow, Queen Victoria's anaesthetist, was so incited by his belief that cholera was water-borne that he wrenched off the handle from the public pump in Broad Street, Soho. The cholera stopped. (Like the best medical stories, this was invented by his biographer. Snow explained modestly that the mortality fell because everyone had fled. So impressive a public health measure, even if fictitious, in 1955 bestowed John Snow's name upon the local pub, probably to the spiritual ire of so rabid a teetotaller.)

There was another Public Health Act in 1872: 343 sections of it, creating pure water, flushed sewers, clean streets, healthy dwellings, rubbish tips, food inspectors, tidy markets and burial under the most sanitary conditions. The volume of opinion swelled, that there should be laws against us naturally filthy humans infecting each other. A surgeon to the Sunderland Eye Infirmary, Reginald Orton (1810–62), extended his practice to force repeal of the window tax in 1851 (he also invented the lifeboat). The health visitor was born in 1888, to instruct mothers how to look after babies. The 1900s regulated midwives, factories and children, and compelled notification of births and infectious diseases. In 1904, a depressing Committee on Physical Deterioration was inflicted on British schools, inspired by the Boer War generals' outrage at discovering that half their recruits were unfit to fight. After 1916, you could legally demand to have your clap treated anonymously. The USA was meanwhile as vigorously sanitising the thickly arriving huddled masses.

Politicians have now leapt joyfully into the environment. Its trouble is double:

- Increasing CO_2 from oil and coal outruns its normal absorption by our decreasing vegetation. This damages the earth's atmosphere so that heat from sun cannot get out again.
- Fluoride compounds from refrigerators and aerosols destroy the O_3 in the atmosphere's ozone layer. This lets in the sun's ultraviolet rays and gives people skin cancer and cataracts.

To combat all this, we fill up with unleaded and renounce spraying aerosols on our furniture and armpits. Equally reckless contaminators of the atmosphere as our cars' exhaust-pipes are our own. A cow contributes richly to the greenhouse effect by emitting 200 litres of methane gas rearwards a day. Us 5.3 billion humans are less flatulent, but vastly outnumber the cows. Were I an idealistic green-eyed politician, my slogan would be: 'Save the world! Fart in a condom!'

Lies, Damned Lies and Statistics

William Farr (1807–83) studied medicine in Paris and spent his life in our Registrar General's office; his *Vital Statistics* in 1837 gave medicine an invisible instrument as potent as the microscope. A nation's births, marriages and deaths can reveal to a statistician much to penetrate and prevent a nation's ills. Such arithmetic incites widespread mistrust. Miss Nightingale wagged her finger: 'To understand God's thoughts we must study statistics, for these are the measure of his purpose.' Professor Theodor Billroth (1829–94) of Vienna, the first surgeon to remove the stomach, snorted: 'Statistics are like women, mirrors of purest virtue and truth, or like whores, to use as one pleases.' The public shrugs them off: 'Oh, you can prove anything by statistics.' But only to people who cannot understand statistics.

'Fog everywhere. Fog up the river, where it flows among green aits and meadows; fog down the river, where it rolls defiled among the tiers of shipping . . .' The noontime linkman had surrendered to the early-lit gas, but the pea-souper still clogged the London streets, mingling with the trapped smoke from myriad chimney-pots and penetrated by their black snowfall of soot. *Bleak House* needed rewriting only in 1956, after the Clean Air Act. This was inspired by a four-day Dickensian 'London particular' in December 1952, which killed 4,000 people with bronchitis. The deaths in England and Wales from bronchitis in 1952 were 27,268; in 1987 they were 9,821, a rewarding diminution of 17,447. But the public kept the statistics in line by performing their personal polluting, to raise the deaths from cancer of the lung from 14,218 in 1952 to 35,128 in 1987, a persevering over-correction of 20,910.

Bunyan's fearsome 'Captain of all these men of death' is no longer consumption, but cancer. The discovery in 1950 of a sure safeguard against a deadly form of it – and against attack by the Captain's comrades cardiac ischaemia, high blood pressure, gangrene of the legs, and bronchitis – was clearly an occasion for dancing in the hospital forecourts and wine free on prescription. In reality, the public objected surlily. They did not believe in statistics. Their arguments blew out like a mouthful of smoke: it's too late now to stop, my ninety-year-old grandpa smokes forty a day, I should only put on weight, and who wants to live for ever? Our politicians sat on their hands, or wrung them, or extended them to the tobacco companies; who are perfectly entitled to make their shareholders money, but not to use it evilly to deny and decry a life-saving medical discovery before an audience of eager disbelievers.

What is health? 'A state of complete physical, mental and social well-being and not merely the absence of disease or infirmity,' defines the World Health Organisation. Which is unstatistical, but as helpful as asserting that happiness is achievable only in Heaven.

The National Health

The British National Health Service was founded by Bismarck. The Iron Chancellor, the dropped pilot of Sir John Tenniel's evergreen 1890 *Punch* cartoon, pushed through a difficult Reichstag between 1883 and 1889 laws which created insurance schemes for illness, for accidents from the proliferating machinery, and for chronic invalidism among the workers of Wilhelm I's new German Empire. The world knew nothing like it. A hundred years later, the world had something like it almost everywhere. 'Give the worker the right to work, as long as he is still healthy. Look afer him when he is ill. Take care of him when he is old,' said Bismarck as admirably as Keir Hardie.

Bismarck established *Ortskrankenkassen*, local sickness insurance funds, two-thirds financed and entirely controlled by the workers, which paid the doctors and chemists direct. Before descending Kaiser Bill's pilot's ladder, Bismarck was pronouncing his Social Insurance to be a finer German achievement even than his country's hailed unification in 1871. He was convinced that the prospect of an old age pension would keep the workers contentedly in their places for ever.

Chancellor of the Exchequer in Asquith's 1908 Liberal Government was Lloyd George (1863–1945). 'The People' were as close to his heart as were 'the Dukes' to his damnation. His first budget in 1909 was predictably 'the People's', and equally so it was indigestible by the dukes' noble friends in the House of Lords. They spewed it up, to cause the general election of 14 January 1910, before which Lloyd George sensibly took a breather on the Côte d'Azur.

Lloyd George had dispatched a junior Treasury Civil Servant, W. J. Braithwaite (1875–1938), a clergyman's son who became an expert on income tax, to tour Germany and discover how Bismarck had done it all. On the Tuesday morning of 3 January 1911, Mr Braithwaite arrived on the overnight express at Nice. Lloyd George invited him to join a few friends on the pier, and over drinks heard him talk for four hours (they had prudently distanced themselves from the pier band). In the famed Riviera winter sunshine, above the tideless and still sanitary Mediterranean, possibly over Pernod and little black olives, was conceived the National Health Insurance Act of 1911, which grew up to be the National Health Service Act of 1946. There is no pier at Nice, but A. J. P. Taylor, who tells the enviable story, feels that makes it an even better one.

The People's health was to Lloyd George a solemn item which he intended to evangelise. Before Lloyd George, the voting potential of health had been overlooked. Starvation brought revolution, but sickness was a private misery beyond political remedy. Lloyd George's discovery created the modern cult of mass health care, contemporaneous with mass transport, mass advertising and mass entertainment.

Naturally, some hale and kindly humans had always suffered qualms about the ill ones. Those sitting in Parliament in 1834 amended the Poor Laws to create sick wards in the workhouses for local paupers to die in. Private benefactors subscribed richly to the ancient voluntary hospitals like Guy's or Thomas's or St Bartholomew's, which was established by the monk Rahere in 1123 and refounded by Henry VIII for the sick poor, who were becoming such a dreadful nuisance in the City streets. Hospital entrance halls round the country are thick with names which won immortality by donations, often on quite reasonable terms, and it is sad that socialism arrogantly removed charity from medicine in the NHS. There would be no more Flag Days, with pretty nurses rattling tins.

There was a painful fissure between these proud hospitals, where the doctors applied their learning free and the nurses their devotion for little, and the workhouses where you languished in humble hope. The voluntary hospitals could pick their patients, favouring the interesting few acute before the many lingering chronic. With bumbling British traditionalism, this gap persisted between the voluntary and municipal hospitals until the red-streaked dawn of the NHS.

Doctors before Lloyd George were already in the pay of friendly societies like the Oddfellows or the Druids, or they were hired by union lodges, collieries and the railways, or they ran their own health clubs (the canvassers got 25 per cent commission). A half-a-crown a year sub brought good value to the patient and local esteem to the doctor – except from the insistent bottle-a-week medicine consumer, the trade unionist who enjoyed treating him as an employee, and the wife who enjoyed commanding him as a servant. A few of the greedy and the graceless are eternal in every medical practice.

Lloyd George determined to outdo the Germans. He offered the electorate 'ninepence for fourpence', which sounded a good bargain. All weekly wage earners under £3 paid 4d, their employers 3d, the State 2d, towards the six shillings a year awarded the doctor. The Germans had contributed 9d, and had to pay for the first three days of illness, which in Britain came free. Bismarck gave six weeks' maternity benefit, but Lloyd George settled for a 30-shilling maternity grant, the British not considering pregnancy a disorder. Unpregnant wives, children and the self-employed were left uncovered, though private health insurance was allowed. Both the British and the German payments were compulsory, they were deductible from wages, and involved the post office, cards and stamps. There was respectful confusion in England at duchesses having to affix their maids'.

Professional Opinions

The doctors objected violently. Medical mass meetings were held in Manchester and London's Queen's Hall, where they sang 'Rule Britannia'. Doctors said the unwilling patient would be bullyingly allotted his doctor by the Government, which was unethical; also, it would ruin private practice. Blackleg doctors were rumoured bussed in from Scotland. Unhealthy foreigners were reported swarming across the Channel for free treatment on the British taxpayer. Panel patients were later claimed to be dropping dead through doctors' overwork, and they certainly got no fires in their winter waiting-rooms. The fuss usefully projected the doctors on to the controlling committees, and won them more money. Like most British fuss, it died down. 'The doctors licked their wounds and the duchesses licked their stamps,' concluded E. S. Turner.

The Ministry of Health established in 1919 was a floppy bureaucratic bundle of local government and health insurance business, which mitigated its shortcomings by creating a Consultative Council sweepingly to plan the betterment of the nation's health. Major-General Dawson RAMC had been lecturing a lot about this, and once demobbed was conscripted as chairman. He swiftly became Lord Dawson, and later killed the King. He also thought Hitler rather a good chappie, and that the unemployed should have compulsory physical jerks.

The Dawson report of 1920 outlined a health service comprehensive from professors to pharmacists. There would be 'primary health centres' with beds for GPs to treat their patients, and 'secondary health centres' for consultants when they failed to get better. Infectious and mental diseases would be locked away on their own, and everyone would have a medical record-card. Doctors would run the show, as soldiers and sailors ran the Army and Navy ('The practice of putting the skilled under the unskilled must cease,' was one way of regarding the Civil Service).

The Dawson blueprint was pencilled across in varying

political shades. Neville Chamberlain (1869–1940) became Minister of Health in 1924, pushed twenty-one reforming bills through Parliament in four years, and abolished the overspending local boards of guardians who applied the poor laws, which were clumsily muddled up with the medical ones. In World War Two, with the admirable spirit which began planning D-Day at Dunkirk, the enduring health and happiness of the British people was studied intensively. The Beveridge Report of 1942 postulated a National Health Service. The Report reflected either an overdue rectification of social injustice long suffered by the British people, or a tardy recognition of their enduring belief that all the unpleasant things in life – sickness, education, unemployment, pensions, tap-water, roads, dustmen, trains, museums, policemen, funerals – should be paid for by Someone Else. That Someone Else was always Them in the end never caught public imagination.

Continued deep concern for the nation's health was useful in winning Labour the 1945 election, and another Welshman brought another health scheme. The doctors objected violently.

Nye Bevan (1897–1960) fixed everything with Corkscrew Charlie and Charles Hill (1904–1989), the secretary of the BMA, who was famous also as the 'Radio Doctor' of rich phraseology (like 'little black-coated workers', when he meant prunes). Nye Bevan saw that the way to medical care for all regardless of its expense was 'stopping the consultants' mouths with gold'. Two fossils of 1948 are as alive and as succulent today as newly-opened Whistables.

The magic number '9/11ths' in consultants' contracts means that nine of the eleven half-days of each working week (in Nye Bevan's time everyone worked on Saturday mornings, if you can believe it) shalt thou labour for an NHS salary; but thou can do as much private practice as feasible during the remaining 2/11ths, which include Sunday, every evening, early morning, and far into the night if you are sufficiently energetic or rapacious. Nye's other golden gob-stopper was a 'merit award', given secretly by your medical peers, and adding to both your pay and your pension. Any City company awarding its directors with similar discreet generosity would face a turbulent shareholders' annual meeting, followed by arrival of the fraud squad.

The NHS was inaugurated on Monday 5 July 1948, to miners' brass bands at dawn playing 'O Happy Morn'. It had already been running efficiently for nine years.

Between 3 September and 3 November 1939, the British Government expected 600,000 dead and 1,200,000 wounded in air raids. The Ministry of Health needed 3,000,000 hospital beds at once. (The entire wartime toll was 60,000 dead and 235,000 wounded, though until the easing of the Blitz in 1941 more British civilians were killed than British servicemen.) The Government thus inaugurated the Emergency Medical Service, with the Minister of Health its dictator and paymaster. The EMS effectively owned all British Hospitals, and duplicated potentially bombed ones with prefabricated wards and operating theatres sprawling across green fields, while special centres were created for chest, brain, limb and plastic surgery, the blood-transfusion service was nationalised, the pathology service rationalised, and Victorian 'asylums' were transformed into busy teaching hospitals. The Canadians then the Yanks erected their own lavish military hospitals, which stayed to succour their hosts.

The only fundamental change from the EMS to the NHS was the abolition of Lloyd George's GP panel system. As the fundamental difference between the wartime state and the welfare one was only the welcome absence of bombs.

'The desire to take medicine is perhaps the greatest feature that distinguishes man from animals,' mused Sir William Osler. Nobody else had noticed this. The British genius is an infinite capacity for taking pills. From the 1949 newspapers, the whole country was demanding free teeth, glasses, wigs and artificial legs, with spares. Nye Bevan imagined that free treatment would turn the voters so healthy so rapidly that the medical services would wither away, like the state in Engels' imagination of communism. Such unworldliness implies that Bevan really reached his peak as a union official in South Wales.

The biggest boon of the NHS, like professional nursing emerging from the Crimean War, was unexpected. Hospitals became humane. The patient's disease was no longer considered the property of the consultant. He was no longer chillily admitted, had his clothes taken away, was confined to bed and bedpans, then one morning laid by two strange men on a trolley and wheeled to another who stifled him, and a few days later handed his clothes back and evicted to the bus queue. Patients daring to ask questions won the consultant's benevolent response: 'Your disease has got a long Latin name, which you wouldn't understand, anyway.'

Food was now prepared as if somebody was necessitated to eat it. The wards lost their Pentonville starkness and discipline. 'At the foot of every bed, confronting its moribund occupant, was a television box. Television was left on, a running tap, from morning to night,' wrote Aldous Huxley in 1932, and the NHS soon caught up with *Brave New World*.

Most nations' health schemes reflect their medical attitudes. Under the British one, the private patient pays to avoid waiting, and the NHS patient waits to avoid paying. The Canadians regulate the fees for doctors and hospitals and repay the patient most of them. The Americans provide for the social substratum and let the rest, or their employers, buy its own health insurance. A Canadian costs twice as much, an American almost three times, to keep healthy than a Briton. The NHS gives good value for less money, because it has no option.

Lloyd George had proclaimed in 1909, 'This is a war budget, for raising money to wage implacable warfare against poverty and squalidness.' In 1960, Enoch Powell made 'the unnerving discovery that every minister of health makes at or near the onset of his term of office, that the only subject he is ever destined to discuss with the medical profession is money'. Better health – well, better health services – means higher taxes, politically the road to Beachy Head.

The National Health Service, like the car made on a Friday afternoon, needed repairs from the start. Its committees of enquiry bear our greatest postwar names: Guillebaud, Maud, Porritt, Gillie, Cranbrook, Bonham-Carter, Salmon, Seebohm, Robinson, Crossman, Castle, Powell and, er, Cogwheel. The NHS was reformed in 1974, so effectively that five years later it had to be reformed all over again. Since then, it has been reformed as it goes along, depending on what reads worst in the papers any morning. In 1990 the Government decided it should be *properly* reformed. It would become a fee-paying service for private patients, except that nobody paid anything. The doctors objected violently.

'Never was legislation more needed. Never was it less wanted,' lamented the Minister.

Not the medical mouthpiece of Mrs Thatcher or Mr Major or Mr Kinnock, but Lloyd George in 1911.

The fiery illnesses of youth are extinguished, the smouldering ones of age confined, the easements of life have been ingeniously bettered, multiplied and scattered, the sick recover to fall sick again, the elderly of today are the dead of yesterday.

The intelligent reader will have grasped that the potential of medicine is infinite, the demands on medicine must be unrestrained, but the resources for medicine are limited. Unless a fearless politician strikes a non-political compromise between all three, the history of medicine, like the history of the world in *1066 And All That*, will come to a.

One Small Step for a Man,
One Giant Leap for Mankind

1 The circulation of the blood, expounded to Charles I by William Harvey in 1628, most respectfully.
2 Vaccination against smallpox, hit upon by Edward Jenner in 1796, after that apple-cheeked Gloucestershire milkmaid had enlightened him over the pails: 'Oh, no, sir, but I can't get the smallpox, because you see, I've already had the cowpox.'
3 The theory of evolution in 1859 from Charles Darwin, who spent five highly uncomfortable years sailing the South seas crammed with seventy-three others in the 90-foot long 242 ton *HMS Beagle* to evolve it.
4 Anaesthesia, invented by the pair of New England dentists in the mid-1840s, with the reasonable idea of making a packet out of it.
5 Antisepsis in surgery, devised by Lord Lister with his steam-driven carbolic-spray 'donkey-engine' of 1865.

6 The discovery of microbes by Pasteur, Koch and ranks of orderly-minded Germans in the busy last twenty years of the nineteenth century.

7 Drugs to cure infections, discovered by Gerhard Domagk in the Rhineland the month before Hitler took over in 1933. These were the sulphonamides, which inspired Florey to invent penicillin at Oxford in the year of the Battle of Britain (Fleming had little to do with it).

8 Vitamins, traces in food clinically conspicuous by their absence, perceived by Sir Frederick Gowland Hopkins at Cambridge in 1912.

9 X-rays, accidentally discovered by modest and dreamy Wilhelm Röntgen in Würzburg in 1895, and the matching discovery of radium by Pierre and Marie Curie of Paris and Warsaw 1898.

10 The dominating endocrine glands, mapped in the body between 1854 and 1922 by Claude Bernard of the Sorbonne, who conceived that we had a *milieu intér-ieur*; by Banting and Best of Toronto and insulin; and by Harvey Cushing of Baltimore and the pituitary.

11 Psychiatry – Freud in the 1890s.

12 The configuration of the DNA molccule, the double helix of Crick and Watson of Cambridge in the 1960s, the decade when man began exploring his inner chemistry and outer space.

Of this we may be sure, that science, in obeying the law of humanity, will always labour to enlarge the frontiers of life.

Louis Pasteur,
inaugurating the
Institut Pasteur in 1888.

References

General

Barker, F. & Jackson, P. *The history of London in maps.* London: Barrie & Jenkins, 1990.

Ellis, H. *Bailey and Bishop's notable names in medicine and surgery* (4th edn). London: Lewis, 1983.

Garrison, F. H. *An introduction to the history of medicine* (4th edn). Philadelphia: Saunders, 1929.

Griffith, E. F. *Doctors by themselves.* London: Cassell, 1951.

Guthrie, D. *A history of medicine* (2nd edn). London: Nelson, 1958.

Major, R. H. *Classic descriptions of disease* (3rd edn). Springfield: Thomas, 1945.

Monro, T. K. *The physician as man of letters, science and action* (2nd edn). Edinburgh: Livingstone, 1951.

Turner, E. S. *Call the doctor.* London: Joseph, 1958.

Hippocrates and all That

Clark, K. *Leonardo da Vinci anatomical drawings at Windsor Castle* (2nd edn). London: Phaidon, 1968/69. Vol. 3, 19097.

Huxley, J. *Essays of a biologist* (3rd edn). Harmondsworth: Penguin, 1939.

Keynes, Sir G. *The life of William Harvey.* Oxford: Clarendon Press, 1966.

Scratcherd, T. *Aids to physiology.* Edinburgh: Churchill, 1989.

Man, Microbes and History

Camus, A. *The plague.* London: Hamish Hamilton, 1948.

Dubois, R. J. *Louis Pasteur.* London: Gollancz, 1951.

Homer. *The Iliad.* Tr. E. V. Rieu. Harmondsworth: Penguin, 1950. Book 19.

Thompson, E. S. *Influenza.* London: Percival, 1890.

The Times, 26 August 1988.

The Times, 16 October 1990.

Wells, H. G. *The war of the worlds.* London: Heinemann, 1898.

Zinsser, H. *Rats, lice and history.* New York: Little, Brown, 1935.

Discoveries in the Dark

British National Formulary (No. 16). London: The Pharmaceutical Press, 1988.

Culpeper, N. *The English physitian enlarged.* London: Peter Cole, 1653.

Domagk, G. Ein Beitrang zur Chemotherapie der bakteriellen Infektionen. *Deutsche Medizinische Wochenschrift,* 15 February 1935.

Drummond, J. C., and Wilbraham, A. *The Englishman's food* (2nd edn). London: Cape, 1957.

Fisher, R. B. *Joseph Lister.* London: Macdonald & Jane's, 1977.

Fleming, A. On the antibacterial action of cultures of a penicillium with special reference to their use in the isolation of B. influenzae. *Br. J. Exp. Path*, 1929. 10: 226.

Hare, R. *The birth of penicillin*. London: Allen & Unwin, 1970.

Hörlein, H. The development of chemotherapy for bacterial diseases. *Practitioner*, 1937. 195: 635.

Husband, H. A. *The student's hand-book of forensic medicine and public health* (5th edn). Edinburgh: Livingstone, 1889.

Jenner, E. *An inquiry into the causes and effects of the variolæ vaccinæ*. London: Sampson Low, 1798.

Macfarlane, G. *Howard Florey*. Oxford: University Press, 1979.

Mietzsch, F., Behnisch, R. *Therapeutisch verwendbare Sulfonamid- und Sulfon-Verbindungen* (2nd edn). Weinheim: Verlag Chemie GmbH, 1955.

Smith, J. R. *The speckled monster*. Chelmsford: Essex Record Office, 1987.

The Times, 17 August 1988.

Trials of war criminals before the Nuernberg military tribunals under control council law no. 10. Nuernberg October 1946–April 1949. Washington: 1952. viii, 1091.

The Conquest of Pain

Atkinson, R. S., Rushman, G. B., Lee, J. A. *A synopsis of anaesthesia* (10th edn). Bristol: Wright, 1987.

Duncum, B. M. *The development of inhalation anaesthesia*. Oxford: Oxford University Press, 1947.

Hewer, C. L. *Recent advances in anaesthesia and analgesia* (6th edn). London: Churchill, 1948.

Huysmans, J-K. *À rebours*, 1884.

MacQuitty, B. *The battle for oblivion*. London: Harrap, 1969.

World Medicine, 5 March 1983.

The Gold-headed Cane

Grace, P. First among women. *BMJ* 1991; 303: 1582–3.

Macmichael, M. (3rd edn Munk, W.) *The gold-headed cane*. London: Longmans Green, 1884.

Nightingale, F. *Notes on nursing*. London: Harrison, 1859.

Sayre, A. *Rosalind Franklin and DNA*. New York: Norton, 1975.

Verney, H. *Florence Nightingale at Harley Street*. London: Dent, 1970.

Watson, J. D. *The double helix*. London: Wiedenfeld & Nicolson, 1968.

Weatherall, D. J. *The new genetics and clinical practice*. Oxford: University Press, 1985.

The Demon Barbers

Cowles, V. *Edward VII and his circle*. London: Hamilton, 1956.

Grogono, B. J. S. Changing the hideous face of war. *BMJ* 1991; 303: 1568–8.

McDowell, F. *The source book of plastic surgery*. Baltimore: Williams & Wilkins, 1977.

Medvei, V. C. & Thornton, J. L. *The royal hospital of Saint Bartholomew 1123–1973*. London: St Bartholomew's Hospital, 1974.

Mosley, R. *Faces from the fire*. London: Weidenfeld, 1962.

Pound, R. *Gillies surgeon extraordinary*. London: Joseph, 1964.

Richardson, R. G. *Larrey: surgeon to Napoleon's Imperial Guard*. London: Murray, 1974.

Thornton, J. L. *John Abernethy*. London: Marshall, 1953.

Treves, Sir F. *The elephant man and other reminiscences*. London: British Publishers Guild, 1941.

Sex and its Snags

Bourne, A. W. *A doctor's creed*. London: Gollancz, 1962.
Freyer, P. *The birth controllers*. London: Secker & Warburg, 1965.
Hall, R. *Marie Stopes*. London: Deutsch, 1977.
Harris, F. *My life and loves*. New York: Grove Press, 1963.
Ober, W. B. *Boswell's clap and other essays*. Carbondale & Edwardsville: South Illinois University Press, 1979.
Rolph, C. H. *The trial of Lady Chatterley*. Privately printed, 1961.
The Times, 19, 20 July, 1938.

Dead Ends

Fraser, I. The discards of surgery. *British Medical Journal*, 1963: i, 839–843.
Johnson, J. R. *A treatice on the medicinal leech*. London: Longman, 1816.
Layton, T. B. *Sir William Arbuthnot Lane, Bt*. Edinburgh: Livingstone, 1956.

Odd Practices

Cliford, T. *Cures*. New York: Macmillan, 1980.
Dictionary of national biography 1941–1950. Oxford: University Press, 1959.
Inglis, B., West, R. *The alternative health guide*. London: Joseph, 1983.
Jameson, E. *The natural history of quackery*. London: Joseph, 1961.
Jeafferson, J. C. *A book about doctors*. London: Hurst & Blacket, 1860.
Krumbhaar, E. B. Bath olivers – doctor and biscuit. *Annals of Medical History*, 1929: i, 3, 253–9.
Logan, P. *Making the Cure*. Dublin: Talbot, 1972.
Quackery in the past. *BMJ*, 1911: i, 1250–1263.
Read, W. Some notable quacks. *BMJ*, 1911: i, 1264–1274.

Smollett, T. *An essay on the external use of water.* London: Cooper, 1752.

White, G. *The natural history of Selborne.* 1789. Letter 8 January, 1776.

Freud, the English Governess and the Smell of Burnt Pudding

Jones, E. *The life and work of Sigmund Freud.* London: Hogarth, 1953–57.

Stafford-Clark, D. *What Freud really said.* London: Macdonald, 1965.

Roazen, P. *Freud and his followers.* London: Allen Lane, 1976.

Wollheim, R. *Freud.* London: Fontana, 1971.

Scholars, Truants and Teachers' Pets

Heston, L. L., Heston R. *The medical casebook of Adolf Hitler.* London: Kimber, 1979.

Kershaw, A. *A history of the guillotine.* London: Calder, 1958.

Reid, M. *Ask Sir James.* London: Hodder & Stoughton, 1987.

Treue, W. *Doctor at court.* London: Weidenfeld, 1958.

Watson, F. The death of George V. *History Today,* December 1986.

The Body Politic

Hennock, E. P. *British social reform and German precedents.* Oxford: Clarendon Press, 1987.

Higham, F. M. C. *Lord Shaftesbury.* London: S. C. M. Press, 1945.

Levitt, R. *The reorganised National Health Service.* London: Croom Helm, 2nd edn. 1977.

Ritter, G. A. *Social welfare in Germany and Britain.* Leamington Spa: Berg, 1986.

Taylor, A. J. P. *Bismarck*. London: Hamish Hamilton, 1955.

Taylor, A. J. P. *English history 1914–1945*. Oxford: Clarendon Press, 1965.

Taylor, A. J. P. *Essays in English history*. London: Penguin, 1976.

Trevelyan, G. M. *Illustrated English social history*. London: Longmans, 1944.

Watson, F. *Dawson of Penn*. London: Chatto & Windus, 1950.

Watson, F. *History today*, 25 January 1989.